"You think the battle for real health care reform is over? John Geyman says 'Not on your life!' And, by the way, your life is what's at stake. This former Republican country doctor and long-time respected scholar, editor, and advocate for reform that puts the patient, not the industry, first, has issued an informed, convincing, and passionate account of why the battle has just begun, and how we, the people, can win."

—Bill Moyers, American journalist and public commentat
and author of: *Moyers on Democracy*

"In what may be Dr. Geyman's best book to date, *Hijacked* lays bare the corporate influences that led Congress to its politically compromised version of health care "reform," the Patient Protection and Affordable Care Act of 2010 (PPACA). *Hijacked* shows how this controversial legislation does more for corporate shareholders than it does for patients. But it goes beyond the problems to describe comprehensive approaches to true health care reform."

—Lee Burnett, D.O., Executive Director, The Student Doctor Network

The Good News

On the upside, the new health care "reform" legislation brought forward this impressive list of steps:

- Extending health insurance to 32 million more people by 2019.
- Subsidies to help lower-income people afford health insurance.
- Allowance for parents to keep their children on their policies until age 26.
- Expansion of Medicaid to cover 16 million more lower-income Americans
- $11 billion of new funding for community health centers that could enable them to nearly double their current patient volume.
- Coverage without cost-sharing of preventive services recommended by the U.S. Preventive Services Task Force, together with an annual wellness visit with a personalized prevention plan.
- Phasing out by 2020 the "doughnut hole" coverage gap for the Medicare prescription drug benefit.
- Creation of a new voluntary national insurance program for long-term services: Community Living Assistance Services and Supports (CLASS) program.
- Creation of a non-profit Patient-Centered Outcomes Research Institute charged with examining the relative outcomes, clinical effectiveness and appropriateness of different medical treatments.
- Initiating some limited reforms of the insurance industry, including prohibition of pre-existing condition exclusions and banning of annual and lifetime limits.
- Providing a 10 percent bonus for primary care physicians, together with some provisions to expand the primary care workforce.

The Bad News

On the downside, the new health care "reform" law will fail to remedy uncontrolled costs, inadequate access to affordable health care, widespread health disparities, and variable quality of care:

- Surging costs of health care will not be contained.
- Uncontrolled costs of health care and insurance will make them unaffordable for a large and growing part of the population.
- The new bill will fall far short of universal coverage.
- Quality of care for the U.S. population is unlikely to significantly improve.
- Insurance "reforms" are incomplete and will be largely ineffective.
- New layers of waste and bureaucracy, without added value, will further fragment our system.
- Costs of the new bill are projected only for *government* spending, missing the point of what patients and families will be forced to pay.
- With its lack of price controls, the new bill will prove to be a bonanza for corporate stakeholders in the medical-industrial complex.
- Perverse incentives within an unregulated market-based system will still lead to overtreatment with inappropriate and unnecessary care while millions of Americans forego necessary care because of cost.
- The "reformed" system is not sustainable and will require more fundamental reform down the road to rein in the excesses of the market.

Also by John Geyman, M.D.

Family Practice: Foundation of Changing Health Care

Family Practice: An International Perspective in Developed Countries
(Co-Editor)

Evidence-Based Clinical Practice: Concepts and Approaches (Co-Editor)

Textbook of Rural Medicine (Co-Editor)

Health Care in America: Can Our Ailing System Be Healed?

The Corporate Transformation of Health Care:
Can the Public Interest Still Be Served?

Falling Through the Safety Net: Americans Without Health Insurance

Shredding the Social Contract: The Privatization of Medicare

The Corrosion of Medicine: Can the Profession Reclaim its Moral Legacy?

Do Not Resuscitate: Why the Health Insurance Industry is Dying,
and How We Must Replace It

The Cancer Generation: Baby Boomers Facing a Perfect Storm

HIJACKED

THE ROAD TO SINGLE PAYER IN THE AFTERMATH OF STOLEN HEALTH CARE REFORM

John Geyman, M.D.

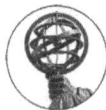

Copernicus Healthcre
Friday Harbor, WA

Hijacked: The Road to Single Payer
sin the Aftermath of Stolen Health Care Reform

Book design, cover and illustrations by Bruce Conway
Author photograph by Anne Sheridan

ISBN paper: 978-1-938218-09-5
ISBN ebook: 978-1-56751-403-2

Library of Congress Cataloging-in-Publication Data
is available from publisher on request.

Coperncicus Healthcare
Friday Harbor, WA
www.copernicus-healthcare.org

First printing
Printed by CreateSpace in the U.S.A.

- the families of the 45,000 Americans who die each year without health insurance
- the 2,000,000 cancer patients who forego medical services each year due to unaffordable costs
- the tens of millions who will be underinsured even after the health care "reform" law of 2010
- the greater number of Americans who remain just one accident or major illness away from personal and family disaster
- American business, large and small, which finds itself less competitive in global markets and unable to afford the crushing burden of health care costs, and
- to physicians and other health professionals who encounter increasing bureaucratic obstacles to providing the kind of care they want to provide.

There is a better way, as a majority of Americans have known for some 60 years, and as this book lays out. May the day dawn when all Americans gain access to necessary health care as their birthright, joining citizens of most other advanced countries around the world where professionalism and care outweigh commercialism and profiteering on the backs of sick people.

Contents

Tables and Figures

Acknowledgments

This book would not have been possible without the help of many. I am indebted to these colleagues for their constructive comments and suggestions through their peer review of selected chapters:

- Larry Green, M.D., Epperson-Zorn Chair for Innovation in Family Medicine at the University of Colorado, Denver
- Ida Hellander, M.D., Executive Director of Physicians for a National Health Program (PNHP), Chicago
- Don McCanne, M.D., past president of Physicians for a National Health Program and PNHP Senior Health Policy Fellow
- John Nyman, Ph.D., Professor of Health Services Research and Policy, University of Minnesota
- Roger Rosenblatt, M.D., MPH, Professor of Family Medicine, University of Washington, Seattle
- John Saultz, M.D., Professor and Chairman, Department of Family Medicine, Oregon Health Sciences University, Portland
- Gayle Stephens, M.D., Professor Emeritus of Community and Family Medicine, University of Alabama at Birmingham School of Medicine
- Robert Stone, M.D., emergency physician in Bloomington, Indiana and Director of Hoosiers for a Commonsense Health Plan
- Andrew Wilper, M.D., internist and Associate Director of the University of Washington Internal Medicine Residency Program in Boise, Idaho

I am also indebted to many investigative journalists, health professionals and others who have dared to confront and expose the business practices of health care industries that run counter to the public interest. Reports of many organizations have been helpful in fleshing out what really goes on in health care, including those of the Center for National Health Program Studies, the Center for Public Integrity, the Center for Responsive Politics, the Center for Studying Health System

Change, the Commonwealth Fund, Fairness & Accuracy in Reporting (FAIR), the Kaiser Family Foundation, the National Academy of Social Insurance, the Pew Center for the People and the Press, Physicians for a National Health Program and Public Citizen. Various government reports have been especially useful, including those of the Medicare Payment Advisory Commission (MEDPAC), the Centers for Medicare/ Medicaid Services (CMS), the Congressional Budget Office (CBO), and the General Accounting Office (GAO). I also thank the publishers and journals that granted permission to reprint or adapt materials as cited throughout the book. Special thanks to Matt Wuerker of *Politico* and John Trever of the *Albuquerque* Journal for generously allowing reprinting of their insightful cartoons.

I am especially grateful to Greg Bates, publisher at Common Courage Press, for his encouragement and support through this and my previous five books. He is also a rigorous and insightful editor who again makes this book better than it would otherwise have been.

Bruce Conway of Illumina Publishing, Friday Harbor, Washington brought his many skills to book design, cover and interior layout, preparation of all graphics, typesetting, and making the book available in ebook form. Andrew Seltser in Friday Harbor proofed the entire manuscript with his professional eye. Carolyn Acheson of Edmunds, Washington with her long experience in indexing, created a reader-helpful index for the book.

As with all my previous books, I am most of all indebted to Gene, my wife, partner and soul mate over these 54 years, who has helped in so many ways to make this work possible.

PREFACE

The Health Care Boondoggle: An Unforeseen Boon
to the Single Payer Movement

"Americans will always do the right thing—after they exhaust all the alternatives."

—Winston Churchill

Is Health Care "Reform" 2010 better than nothing? After a protracted political battle that filled media news cycles for over 15 months, a comprehensive bill for health care "reform" was enacted in the United States. In late March 2010, the Health Care and Education Affordability Reconciliation Act of 2010 (H.R. 4872) was passed by Congress and signed into law by President Obama. The outcome of this legislation was uncertain until the final votes were counted—a cliffhanger all the way.

This new law was immediately hailed by its supporters as an "historic breakthrough" of the magnitude of Social Security, Medicare and Medicaid, and the civil rights movement. At its signing ceremony, President Obama declared:

"After a century of striving, after a year of debate, after a historic vote, health-care reform is no longer an unmet promise. It is the law of the land."[1]

Earlier, after this bill had cleared the Senate, Majority Leader Harry Reid (D-NV) had made similar comments:

"The American people have waited for this moment for a century. This, of course, is a health bill. But it is also a jobs bill, an economic recovery bill, a deficit-reduction bill, an antidiscrimination bill. It is truly a bill of rights. And now it is the law of the land."[2]

But the bill we got is not an historic breakthrough. It is a boondoggle from start to finish. It is a sad reminder of the corrupting influence of money and corporate power in America, ending up as a bonanza for the industries that themselves are the main reason for uncontrolled prices and costs of health care, in turn leading to declining access and variable quality of care, our three biggest system problems. As with the banking industry, the very people and interests that were causing our crisis were asked to fix it, and we are getting what we deserve—a bailout for those interests at our expense. This is far from the reform we urgently need, and will not work.

The hype about this "reform" bill is a lie intended to mollify its critics and make it appear that the hard-fought campaign was a strategic victory that will propel the Democrats to success in the November elections. But this bill is based on continued and increasing subsidies of a dying private insurance industry that would soon be gone if forced to compete with not-for-profit public financing on a level playing field. The bill will be ineffective in reining in health care costs because to do so would have gored the oxen of the stakeholders—*our* cost containment is *their* profits and revenues. Health policy science and the experience of many other advanced countries around the world have been completely ignored by the political class and the media throughout the political process.

Most of us are by now fatigued out by the constant battle over health care reform and all the twists and turns of legislative proposals. But the health care crisis does not go away with the passage of this bill. This is about our health, our lives and our money as patients, families and taxpayers. This is about one of our fellow Americans dying every 12 minutes—45,000 a year for lack of health insurance.[3] They are our friends and neighbors, impacting nearly all lower-income Americans and an increasing number of the middle class. This is about our future and what kind of a country we are, so we all have a big stake in what comes next.

If you are among the many millions of Americans who still believe that markets can fix our problems, that health care corporations have our best interests at heart, that all our elected leaders are devoted to the public interest more than their own self-interest in winning the next election, that the media are generally credible and accurate, that the flaws of the present system will work themselves out over time, or that we will surely get needed reforms if we just elect the right people, then get ready for a rude awakening.

This is a tough story. It is all about power and self-interest, not common sense or logical problem solving. It is not a right-wing conspiracy, just the ongoing havoc wreaked by application of an unfettered business model to health care. It is about hypocrisy of the political class, amounting to legislative malpractice. In short, we have been sold down the river by our political leaders, and are being taken to the cleaners by the continued greed of corporate stakeholders, their allies and surrogates.

If all that seems outlandish and over the top, buckle up and get ready for a wild ride. This is a fully documented factual account of how this bill was made in the Congressional sausage factory. As Paul Harvey used to say: "The truth is stranger than fiction."

As this book reveals, this will be just one more failed attempt in a long string of failures. The battle over health care reform will necessarily erupt again, sooner rather than later. We are all entitled to our own opinions, but not our own facts. By the end of this book, I challenge you to still think that we have the best health care system in the world or that this reform attempt will work if we just give it enough time.

Part I looks at what happened in the 2009-2010 reform attempt, and how the special interests interacted with the political process and hijacked the reform agenda, even while posturing their qualified support. We trace the development of bills in Congress and the tortuous path to the narrow passage of the final bill, drawing from history to place these events in perspective. In Part II we examine the "reform" bill in detail, assessing not only its strengths but also its many shortcomings that will doom it to overall failure. We consider the lessons we can draw from this failure of health policy, update the new realities, and project what we can expect over the next ten years in health care. In Part III we lay out a road map for future reform and show how we can succeed the next time around.

My previous books over the last nine years have dealt with our overall health care system,[4] its transformation by corporate interests,[5] the uninsured and our fragile safety net,[6] the privatization of Medicare,[7] the corrosion of medicine by business interests,[8] the failure and obsolescence of the insurance industry,[9] and the crisis facing baby boomers with cancer as they confront our deteriorating health care system.[10] This book reveals how far we still are from real health care reform, and charts new directions as to how we can reform our market-based system so that it can meet the needs of all Americans.

John P. Geyman, M.D.

July 2010

References

1. Meckler, L, Hitt, G. Obama signs landmark health bill. *Wall Street Journal*, March 26, 2010:A4.
2. Herszenhorn, DM, Pear, R. Final votes in Congress cap battle over health. *New York Times*, March 26, A15. 2010.
3. Wilper, AP, Woolhandler, S, Lasser, K et al. Health insurance and mortality in U.S. adults. *Am J Public Health* 99, 2009.
4. Geyman, JP. *Health Care in America: Can Our Ailing System Be Healed?* Woburn, MA: Butterworth-Heinemann, 2002.
5. Geyman, JP. *The Corporate Transformation of Health Care: Can the Public Interest Still Be Served?* New York: Springer Publishing Company, 2004.
6. Geyman, JP. *Falling Through the Safety Net: Americans Without Health Insurance.* Monroe, ME: Common Courage Press, 2005.
7. Geyman, JP. *Shredding the Social Contract: The Privatization of Medicare.* Monroe, ME: Common Courage Press, 2006.
8. Geyman, JP. *The Corrosion of Medicine: Can the Profession Reclaim Its Moral Legacy?* Monroe, ME: Common Courage Press, 2007.
9. Geyman, JP. *Do Not Resuscitate: Why the Health Insurance Industry is Dying, and How We Must Replace It.* Monroe, ME: 2008.
10. Geyman, JP. *The Cancer Generation: Baby Boomers Facing a Perfect Storm.* Monroe, ME, 2009.

PART I

We Voted for Change—What Happened?

Backroom Politics Behind the
Curtain of "Yes We Can"

CHAPTER 1

"Yes We Can" Meets Machiavelli: Shifting Corporate "Alliances" For and Against Reform

"Change has come. This is our moment. This is our time… to reclaim the American Dream and reaffirm that fundamental truth – that out of many, we are one; that while we breathe, we hope, and where we are met with cynicism, and doubt, and those who tell us that we can't, we will respond with that timeless creed that sums up the spirit of a people: yes, we can."

—Barack Obama on election night 2008[1]

"There is nothing more difficult to take in hand, more perilous to conduct, or more uncertain in its success, than to take the lead in the introduction of a new order of things."

—Niccolò Machiavelli, *The Prince*[2]

Now that health care reform has become law, what do advocates of single payer do next? First, we need to understand what we have just been through, and where the new legislation is taking us. The battle for health care reform since President Obama took office reveals a great deal about the nature of American politics, about the limits of forging consensus, and contains valuable insights for those strategizing to win single payer. We have lived the details exhaustively. Yet certain vignettes and features stand out as particularly instructive.

To understand the political process and outcomes of reform initiatives more clearly, leading policy analyst and scholar in government affairs Mark Peterson offers a powerful lens through which to view competing interests: *Stakeholders* benefit from the status quo, and *stake challengers* do not benefit or are harmed by the status quo.[3] This view reveals an alarming fact about the "reform" just passed: all of the key players are stakeholders—they are invested in the status quo and have sought ways that will enlarge their profits within it. The stake challengers, those who need something different, are patients and American families everywhere. They had no place at the negotiating table. And, as will be made clear, their plight is the core reason why we must keep pressing for a single payer health care system similar to those in many democracies around the world.

PLEDGES, GAMES AND THE QUEST
FOR THE PROFIT GRAIL

In May 2009, President Obama held a high-profile event in the White House, convening leaders from the health care industry to a meeting to discuss reform of the U.S. health care system. Participants included representatives from the insurance, drug, medical device and hospital industries as well as business, labor and organized medicine. This "alliance" for health care reform produced a *voluntary* commitment to reduce the costs of health care by 1.5 percent, which would amount to some $1 trillion over the next 10 years. Participants promised to "cut both overuse and underuse of health care by aligning quality and efficiency initiatives." The White House was quick to call the meeting "an historic day, a watershed event, because these savings will help to achieve comprehensive health care reform."[4]

Indeed, the forces for changing health care seemed on the surface to be perfectly lined up: Democrats controlled both houses of Congress with a filibuster-proof majority in the Senate, and the Executive Branch was in the hands of the most eloquent, diplomatic and popular president in half a century.

Even as partisan and internecine battles among stakeholders reached new levels as members of Congress went home to hear impassioned protests from many constituents, President Obama was still seemingly pleased with the level of stakeholder support for health care reform. In a Rose Garden press briefing in July, he stated: "...the fact that we have made so much progress where we've got doctors, nurses, hospitals, even the pharmaceutical industry, AARP, saying that this makes sense to do, I think means that the stars are aligned and we need to take advantage of that."[5]

The downfall from that high point surprised many, and yet was perfectly predictable given the forces at work. Subsequent weeks and months soon showed the "charm offensive" by major stakeholders in our medical-industrial complex to be a sham alliance as their profoundly different interests revealed starkly incompatible agendas.

A quick look at the four major industries lays bare the reasons why building consensus among them was impossible. Because they were allowed to drive reform, the inevitable result is a system that serves their quest for profit first and puts the health of Americans in a distant second place. The interests of the insurance industry, the drug industry, the hospital industry and of organized medicine in the form of the AMA are worth reviewing as a means to understand why going to them to create reform guaranteed failure.

The Insurance Industry, Obama's Big Carrot and Lessons from When It All Went Stale

As the CEO of the industry's trade group, America's Health Insurance Plans (AHIP), Karen Ignagni said that insurance companies "accept the premise that the system is not working today and needs to be reformed."[6] This new-found flexibility seems laudable—at first. The pledge by the insurance industry was simple—if all Americans were required to buy health insurance, the industry would abandon pre-existing conditions as an underwriting principle, accept all applicants for insurance, and stop charging women higher premiums than men. But sick people would continue to pay more for coverage than healthy people.

As the second largest private insurer, UnitedHealth Group even offered up 15 recommendations that could allegedly save $540 billion in federal health care costs over 10 years, including such steps as "providing patients with incentives for going to high-quality, efficient physicians, granting physicians incentives for providing comprehensive and preventive care, and reducing unnecessary care." UnitedHealth's Center for Health Reform and Modernization also attached speculative cost savings in these areas: "...providing nurse practitioners at nursing homes to manage illness and reduce avoidable hospitalizations ($166 billion), using evidence-based care management with preventive care to reduce avoidable hospitalizations ($102 billion), and analyzing claims before they are paid to prevent duplicate billing and other administrative errors ($57 billion)."[7]

Again, laudable. Yet peel away the surface layers and the motivations for their willingness becomes evident. The $540 billion in savings recommendations discussed above would largely be savings for the insurance companies that wouldn't have to pay the money out. Those savings would increase their profit—no wonder they showed enthusiasm!

Just as important was the industry's agenda in this reform. By having nearly all Americans insured, as many as 50 million new enrollees were in play. The reform meant gaining enormous markets from new enrollees in both private and public plans.

That its agenda was more self-serving than supportive of real reform became clear as the industry took to the battlefield on these fronts:

- Vigorously opposing any public option as an effort to bring competition to the market, claiming that it could not be a level playing field and would put them out of business;
- Opposing any controls or caps on premium rates;
- Fighting against any cuts in overpayments to Medicare Advantage plans or attempts to set medical loss ratios too high (the lower they are, the more income insurers gain);
- Lobbying in favor of setting the lowest possible minimal standards for insurance coverage; and
- Launching ad campaigns to tell the public how the industry is doing its part to support health care reform.

The biggest indication that the insurance industry wanted this reform can be seen in Table 1.1[8] which shows the increase in its campaign contributions as the prospect of change grew.

A great deal is at stake for this industry, which has continued to realize high profits despite the recession. As an example, Anthem/WellPoint, the nation's largest insurer, reported fourth-quarter 2009 profits of $2.7 billion, despite losing 1.4 million enrollees in the same year.[9]

Even as many people lost their jobs and health insurance, some insurers continued to post large profits. Despite a continued fall in commercial enrollees, UnitedHealth Group, for example, reported a 155 percent increase in second-quarter earnings for 2009 compared to 2008, largely as a result of strong growth in its Medicare and Medicaid business.[10] High profits continued as UnitedHealth posted a 21 percent rise in first-quarter profits in 2010 while spending about $560 million in sharcholder dividends for the coming year.[11]

TABLE 1.1

Campaign Contributions by Major Insurers

Insurer	2005-2006	2007-2008
Blue Cross/Blue Shield	$2,451,716	$3,125,921
AFLAC	$1,924,335	$2,211,030
UnitedHealth Group	$1,045,877	$1,568,634
Aetna	$674,950	$721,957
AHIP	$510,561	$591,750

Source: Terhune, C, Epstein, K. Why health insurers are winning. *BusinessWeek*. August 17, 2009: 036.

During the August 2009 recess of Congress, lucrative future rewards were being projected for the insurance industry. An in-depth article in *BusinessWeek* had this to say:

"As the health reform fight shifts this month from a vacationing Washington to congressional districts and local airwaves around the country, much more of the battle than most people realize is already over. The likely victors are insurance giants such as UnitedHealth Group, Aetna, and WellPoint. The carriers have succeeded in redefining the terms of the reform debate to such a degree that no matter what specifics emerge in the voluminous bill Congress may send to President Obama this fall, the insurance industry will emerge more profitable. Health reform could come with a $1 trillion price tag over the next decade, and it may complicate matters for some large employers. But insurance CEOs ought to be smiling."[12]

Wall Street, of course, followed the health care debate with intense interest, since the health care industry accounts for one-sixth of our economy. Within hours after the Obama Administration signaled its willingness to consider alternatives to a public plan, trading in United-

Health and WellPoint jumped about three-fold as investors placed new calls and puts. Health insurance stocks were pushed higher despite a triple-digit loss in the broader markets.[13]

Noting the political gulf between House and Senate bills over health care reform, especially the Senate Finance Committee's strong opposition to a public option, AHIP naturally continued to campaign for a bipartisan health reform bill, trusting that the Senate would defend its interests.

This dynamic of defending and enlarging turf under the guise of supporting reform was remarkably consistent through all stages of the legislative struggle for reform. As will become clear, by looking further into the details we are left without doubt: the health care system must be designed by the government in response to the will of its citizens, not in a consensus building charade with the medical-industrial complex.

The insurance industry, like the other three big players—the drug industry, hospitals and organized medicine—and others, expressed qualified support for the concept of health care reform, but *only* to the extent that any final legislation would increase their own profits in a continued market-based system. But when their business interests were threatened by specific provisions in the developing legislation, they would either withdraw their support for reform or express limited "support" while lobbying quietly behind the scenes against the provisions they found onerous. Each group tried to keep its place at the negotiating table (and to stay off the menu!), maneuvered to avoid becoming marginalized, and broke ranks from other stakeholders whenever their mutual interests diverged.

Let's look more closely at the insurance industry's actions as the political process came down to the final votes in Congress to see what they tell us about political power in the health care fight.

Reform was seen as a windfall for the insurance industry with up to 50 million new enrollees in play if a strong individual mandate ever became law. Thus the industry's trade group, AHIP, viewed with alarm any provisions that would weaken that mandate. The list of such weakening provisions grew longer as legislators tried to appease special interests and their lobbyists. At one point, the Senate Finance Committee reduced the penalty for not complying with the mandate. It became clear that many healthier people would likely rather pay a small fine and go without insurance than pay the premiums. Since this would reduce the risk pool as well as potential growth of their markets, insurers pushed back by saying they could no longer honor their pledge for insurance reforms (however limited), further warning that insurance rates would climb out of sight.[14] Meanwhile, they kept lobbying for crucial fine-print provisions that could augment their future profits, such as working to assure the lowest possible actuarial value and medical loss ratio requirements, and securing the most advantageous ratios for variation of premiums by age (e.g. a 4:1 ratio instead of a 2:1 ratio).

Relations with the White House and other "allies" then became much colder. As President Obama and his staff increasingly called out the industry for its exploitive practices, insurers responded in kind. These are examples of what became their new, more confrontational tactics:

- Dissemination of misleading and incorrect information claiming that the industry's average medical loss ratio (MLR) was 87 percent, taking only 13 percent of premium income for marketing, administration and profits. This claim was soon found to be flawed and untrue in a new study by the Senate Commerce Committee. Based on analysis of regulatory filings from the largest insurers, including WellPoint, UnitedHealth Group, Aetna and Cigna, the committee found that the average MLR in the large employer market was 84 percent, 80 percent for small employers, only 74 percent in the individual market, and as low as 66 percent for some plans.[15]
- Blaming legislators (correctly) that the bills in Congress would not do enough to rein in health care costs, while still proclaiming support for "reform."[16]
- Opposing any form of a public option as anti-competitive, stating that it would drive them out of business on a playing field tilted against them.
- Seeking to build support among seniors by spreading fear among those enrolled in Medicare Advantage plans that would be facing elimination of government overpayments. Meanwhile, executives at Humana, which more than doubled its revenues from its subsidized Medicare Advantage plans since 2004, tried to counter their villain image by saying they were just doing

their job and are human too.[17]

- Subtly blaming patients for their (irresponsible) role in seeking out too much care, thus raising the costs for everyone; for example, Regence BlueCross BlueShield launched a major PR campaign using a slick Internet site, social media and billboards to say that consumers are largely responsible for high premiums.[18]

- Releasing a biased report, prepared under contract by PricewaterhouseCoopers, claiming that the Senate Finance Committee bill could increase premiums 18 percent more than they would otherwise rise over the next ten years to an average of nearly $26,000 for families in 2019; the White House countered by saying that features of the bill that could lower consumer costs were ignored by the study.[19,20]

- Pressuring their own employees to become activists opposing the public option and cuts to Medicare Advantage while urging support of higher penalties for individuals not purchasing insurance.[21]

- Joining with the hospital industry and organized medicine against the Medicare buy-in option for people between 55 and 64 years of age, mostly because of concerns over low reimbursement.[22]

- After passage of the merged bill by the Senate, launching a final lobbying campaign to limit fine-print provisions that would threaten the industry's financial bottom line, including restrictive MLRs, excise taxes on insurers, minimal coverage standards, annual caps on patient's out-of-pocket costs, and elimination of lifetime maximal limits on coverage.[23]

- Funneling $10 to $20 million to the U.S. Chamber of Commerce for a series of negative attack ads against the bills making their way through Congress, even as AHIP's Karen Ignagni continued to proclaim the industry's support for reform.[24]

- Exorbitant hikes in premiums in the first two months of 2010, when the individual mandate, if enacted at all, appeared to fall far short of industry's expectations (e.g. increases of 56 percent in Michigan, 39 percent in California, 24 percent in Connecticut, 23 percent in Maine, and 20 percent in Oregon).[25]

The top five insurers in the country rung up $12 billion in profits in 2009 while dropping 2.7 million enrollees.[26]

This description of the insurance industry begs the question: what right did it have to be at the negotiating table? And by what leap of faith did President Obama believe that negotiating with it would produce the changes he promised the American people, namely near-universal access at lower cost?

A closer look at rate increases in California sheds further light on how aggressively the industry was pursuing profits over service. In early 2010 Anthem Blue Cross, a subsidiary of WellPoint, the nation's largest insurer, announced its rate increases (averaging 25 percent with some up to 39 percent), affecting some 700,000 enrollees. A firestorm of protests erupted, both in California and nationally. Under pressure from state regulators, the company agreed to delay the increases for two months while the State launched an investigation. By state law, insurers must spend at least 70 percent of premium income on health care claims (an MLR very generous to insurers). Regulators are only able to enforce rate controls if the insurer fails to do so.[27]

Not to be outdone by Anthem, other California insurers soon announced large premium increases, including Health Net, Aetna and UnitedHealth. Blue Shield of California led the list, with some rate hikes ranging up to 75 percent. Tom Epstein, vice president of Public Affairs for the company, viewed these hikes as "in line with increases from all major insurers on small business health savings plans." But Brad Wing, co-owner of the *San Francisco Advertiser*, which received an increase of 58 percent, said "that money is going right back to the insurance companies."[28]

Beyond large rate increases for policies of less value, California insurers were denying claims at high rates. A recent study by the Institute for Health and Socio-Economic Policy, the research arm of the California Nurses Association (CNA) and the National Nurses Organizing Committee (NNOC), compared denial rates for the seven leading insurers in California for the first and second six-month periods of 2009. Table 1.2 shows these results, including one-quarter of all claims for Anthem Blue Cross. As Geri Jenkins, Co-President of CNA/NNOC, observed:

> "What we see over and over is an arrogant industry that is indifferent to the pain and suffering caused by routine care denials or economic catastrophe prompted by outrageous price gouging. The denials and pricing practices are both motivated by the prime directive that seems to surpass everything else for these companies—squeezing their patients and providers alike for profits and

TABLE 1.2

Claims Denial Rates
by Leading California Insurers
Second half of 2009, compared to the first half of 2009

- PacifiCare - 41.17 percent (up from 39.6 percent for the first six months of 2009)
- Cigna - 35.43 percent (up from 32.7 percent)
- HealthNet - 25.82 percent (down from 30 percent)
- Kaiser Permanente - 26.96 percent (down from 28.3 percent)
- Anthem Blue Cross - 24.5 percent (down from 27.9 percent)
- Aetna - 6.4 percent (no change)
- Blue Shield - 22 percent (Blue Shield had previously not reported separate denial data, and only began reporting after the media reports on denials)

For the reporting period of July 1, 2009 to December 31, 2009, the denials average 26.05 percent by the seven insurers.

Source: Press release, California Nurses Association. RNs praise Atty Gen. move to subpoena insurance plans. Move follows nurses report on patient claims data denials—NEW DATA—Denial rates averaged 26 percent even after public uproar. Sacramento, CA, February 25, 2010.

revenues regardless who gets hurt along the way."[29]

Meanwhile Anthem, while increasing its premium rates, was marketing new products, so-called *"downgrade options,"* promoting more affordable premiums but with high cost-sharing for stripped-down benefits. One of its new CoreGuard plans, as an example, has a $20,000 annual deductible for a family for in-network services and a separate $20,000 deductible for out-of-network services. Enrollees are also on the hook for an additional $15,000 for co-payments for non-network services and another $4,500 in prescription drug costs, thereby amounting to a potential $59,500 in out-of-pocket expenses for a family, even without considering the costs of drugs not on the formulary and maternity services![30]

Most of us have either personally struggled or know people who have struggled to get insurance companies to pay claims, not to drop the insured once they become sick. The excesses of the insurance industry as it pursues profit at the cost of denying care, even to the point of killing people, have been covered in Congressional hearings, on the campaign trail, in the news and even in documentaries.

But a simple truth from these realities seemed to elude policymakers and politicians in 2009 and later: we cannot rely on businesses designed to maximize profit (which is an obligation of every publicly traded company) to design regulations or an entire system that is aimed at protecting the public at the expense of those profits. Adequate health care can only come from a system designed outside the interests of those maximizing their own profits by reducing care. In this context, it becomes easy to see that creating a proper system to provide health insurance can only be done with the insurance industry barred from designing it.

This insight—that consensus in the public interest has not yet been possible—has major strategic implications, a matter which we will revisit frequently throughout the book before developing a plan of action in the final chapters.

We can see similar limitations with the drug industry, as its unbridled drive for profit cuts against the aim of designing a system to deliver health care to every American.

Needle Park Politics: The Drug Industry Pushes its "Historic" Fix

PhRMA's CEO Billy Tauzin was very familiar with politics and the drug industry. The former Republican turned Democratic Congressman from Louisiana had played a leading role as chairman of a House committee in the design and passage of the Medicare Prescription Drug, Improvement and Modernization Act of 2003 (MMA). That bill turned the new prescription drug benefit over to the private sector and prohibited the government from negotiating drug prices, as the Veterans Administration does so effectively. Tauzin then used the revolving door between government, industry and K Street to become CEO of PhRMA and a top lobbyist in Washington, D.C. with a reported salary in the range of $2 million a year. He continued to lobby against price controls of drugs or importation of drugs from Canada or other countries.[31]

It was this same crusader against drug price regulation who forged an agreement with President Obama and Senator Max Baucus, Chairman of the Senate Finance Committee. In it, PhRMA pledged $80 billion toward the costs of health care reform. Though some of the details of this agreement have since become a matter of controversy, two parts of the pledge are widely known: (1) drug companies would give a 50 percent discount to Medicare beneficiaries for the costs of their drugs in the "doughnut hole" (i.e. annual drug costs between $2,700 and $6,100); and (2) drug companies would give higher rebates on the drug costs of people on Medicare and Medicaid. It was estimated that about $30 billion would be expended for these two purposes over the next 10 years, with the other $50 billion being directed to non-specified costs of reform.

This pledge was hailed as an "historic agreement" by the White House and praised by the AARP, but it soon became clear that much of this pledge would not result in savings to the federal government. Further, as pointed out by Charles Butler, a pharmaceutical analyst at Barclays Capital, those discounts wouldn't cost the drug companies much: "Because of the discounts, Medicare beneficiaries are likely to continue filling prescriptions in the doughnut hole, whereas in the past many stopped taking their medications because the drugs were unaffordable to them."[32]

The main point of contention in the weeks after this agreement was whether the quid pro quo for the drug industry was assurance that the government would not pursue negotiation of drug prices. In August, an internal memo obtained by the *Huffington Post* confirmed that the White House and the drug industry lobby secretly agreed to protect drug companies from price controls.[33] It was only after the memo became public that both sides issued conflicting reports in an effort to backtrack from the controversy. But many progressives in Congress felt betrayed. In response, Speaker of the House Nancy Pelosi declared that the House was not a party to this agreement. The House Energy & Commerce (E&C) Committee, chaired by Henry Waxman (D-CA), soon passed an amendment to the House bill (H.R. 3200) requiring negotiation of drug prices by the government, and many Democratic leaders called for the drug industry to make a bigger commitment to health care reform.[34]

Despite the lack of transparency in whatever deal was made between PhRMA, the President and Senator Baucus, the drug industry's agenda was crystal-clear: expand its markets through wider insurance coverage and government subsidies, avoid price controls and competition from importation of drugs from other countries, and gain maximal patent protection from generic drug-makers of biotech drugs.

Much as the insurance industry felt more secure in the more conservative Senate, the drug industry also counted on the Senate Finance Committee to roll back provisions in any House bill counter to its interests. PhRMA therefore became an active supporter of a bipartisan approach to health care reform. While not lobbying specifically against the public option, it expressed serious concern over any erosion of employer-sponsored health insurance. It also arrayed its forces in these directions:

- Joining with Families USA, a not-for-profit advocacy group for affordable health care, in a $150 million ad campaign supporting health care reform. This campaign included a re-appearance of Harry and Louise, the fictional couple now on Medicare who played a large part in defeating the Clinton Health Plan in 1993-1994. They told us on major national TV channels, some network news and Sunday talk shows that "a little more cooperation, a little less politics, and we can get the job done this time."[35]
- Teaming up with Families USA to lobby for expanded Medicaid coverage for Americans making up to 133 percent of the federal poverty level ($14,000 a year for individuals). As Tauzin said: "When Families USA and PhRMA can get together, I hope that's a sign to everybody in the House and Senate that we can find common ground, and that the president's call to put party aside and to put ideologies aside and try to find what works is a good call."[36]
- Lobbying against proposals that would prohibit brand-name drug makers from paying generic drug makers to delay marketing of lower-cost generic drugs.
- In the first six months of 2009, PhRMA and Pfizer spent $13.1 and $11.7 million in lobbying, respectively.

It was soon apparent that the initiatives taken by the drug industry that appeared to support reform would please its CEOs and stockholders. These early returns were gained:

- Passage by the Senate Committee on Health, Education, Labor and Pensions (HELP) (by a 16-7 vote) of a provision giving manufacturers of branded biotechnology drugs at least 12 years of patent protection before generic manufacturers can bring such drugs to market (the White House proposed seven years while Henry Waxman wanted five).[37]
- Strong projected annual increases on prescription drug spending.[38]

On one level, the tactic of give and take appeared to be working. From the late spring on, the drug industry was faring well by seeming to support health care reform, having pledged $80 billion toward that task over the next ten years in an agreement with the President and Senate Finance Committee (SFC) chairman Max Baucus. It gained 12 years of patent protection through the SFC bill, much better than the Waxman committee in the House had been willing to give. Was this a fair trade, an $80 billion pledge to cut costs in exchange for 12 more years of patent protection? Investors loved it, pushing stock prices up by five to eight percent on Wall Street between September and October.[39] Such excitement suggests it was better for the industry than for the patient—on balance they would make more money, and drugs would be more expensive. If the patients had gotten the better end of the stick, stock prices for investors would have fallen.

But then the industry was hit with a provision in H.R. 3962 (the House bill) that would have the government negotiate drug prices and add another $60 billion over ten years for new rebates to the government and seniors.

So here again, as with the insurance industry, the question for PhRMA became: should it continue to support reform as its earlier agreements seemed to be unraveling?

It was back to playing both sides of the street, simultaneously supporting and opposing reform as it was unfolding and still hoping that any bill clearing the Senate would remain industry friendly. For example, it launched an advertising blitz through its front group, Americans for Stable Quality Care, promoting health care reform in a dozen states targeting fence-sitting senators with pivotal votes in a final health care bill.[40]

Here are examples of campaigns *against* reform, not entirely clear as to their sponsorship:

- Recruitment of Tony Coelho, former Democratic congressman, to chair the industry-backed group called the Partnership to Improve Patient Care. This coalition soon included representatives from drug makers, biotech and medical device companies, the National Alliance for Hispanic Health, the National Alliance on Mental Illness (NAMI), Easter Seals and 120 other groups. While supporting the concept of comparative effectiveness research, it lobbied for an independent board with industry and patient representatives and *against* using research findings for coverage or reimbursement policies.[41]
- Promoting industry interests through a front group, the NAMI, one of the nation's most influential disease advocacy groups. The drug industry provides about three-quarters of its funding. This group has for years fought against state efforts to limit physicians' freedom to prescribe drugs, especially on such public programs as Medicaid, no matter how expensive or ineffective the drugs might be.[42]

Meanwhile, the industry was busy raising its prices—by 9 percent over the previous year, even in the face of a 1.3 percent decline in inflation (e.g. more than a 18 percent increase for Roche's osteoporosis drug, Boniva, and a 12 percent increase for Merck's asthma drug, Singulair. This increase more than cancelled out the cost of the industry's first-year installment on its ten-year pledge of $80 billion toward health care reform. As it did so, it claimed (as usual) that these price increases were necessary to keep up its innovation through R&D. (Actually, the industry spends two to three times more on marketing than does on R&D.)[43] And as the Senate's merged bill went on to the joint conference committee, PhRMA feared that it would be forced to renegotiate (upwards) its original $80 billion deal made between the President and Senator Baucus' SFC in the spring.[44] The industry was already financing a campaign in many state legislatures to head off cuts in drug prices within an expanded Medicaid program as a means of funding health care reform.[45]

In the first two months of 2010, with health care legislation stalled in Congressional gridlock, a revolt took place among drug-makers forcing Tauzin out of his $2 million a year job as head lobbyist for

PhRMA. Even though he had headed off price controls and importation of drugs from other countries, he was accused of being too eager to bargain away the industry's profits and spending too much on an ad campaign supporting health care reform.[46]

These efforts by drug companies to maximize profit at the expense of patients and tax dollars are well-known. But, as with the insurance company discussion, it is worth following through on the strategic implications. First, when the drug companies hire the regulators who use stints in government as springboards to lucrative industry jobs, the interests of patients and taxpayers are shut out.

Secondly, and just as crucially, it is clear that drug company and insurance company interests run counter to each other. The drug companies don't fight Medicare because it increases their market, as would a public option, as long as it doesn't include the ability of that option to negotiate drug prices. The insurance companies want the opposite, as was made clear in their proposals to save money earlier in the chapter: cut back on care, eliminate the public option, cut back on Medicare to expand their share of the health care dollar.

A third insight is worth noting: can parties with competing objectives forge a consensus? Yes, by enlarging the market for both of them—at the expense of a third party, in this case the American public. By expanding health insurance coverage, insurers make more profit, and by eliminating controls on drug costs, drug companies can also win—with the public losing on both fronts. And, as we will see in later chapters, that is exactly what happened. The American public will lose more in the long run than is yet apparent.

This dynamic of smoothing the path for competing interests to work together can succeed with not just two competing parties but with many, as long as someone else foots the bill. We can see this dynamic compounded by the interests of the private hospitals.

The Hospital Industry: Fueling a Medical Arms Race

As with other competing interests, the hospital industry couched its aims for profit in the language of serving the customer. But as we shall see, the goals of profit and service don't run together seamlessly. As Chip Kahn, leader of the Federation of American Hospitals, says: "The hospitals have been for reform all along, so I see the potential for hospitals and our patients to be big winners in this process."[47] Understanding how the two goals of profits vs. service play out further illuminates our central strategic insight of this chapter: allowing these sectors to pursue their unfettered interests under the guise of compromise and consensus has turned into a disaster for the American public.

Faced with increasing political momentum toward some kind of health care reform, the hospital industry, together with other major stakeholders, wanted to retain its place at the negotiating table and protect its interests in whatever legislation resulted. Urgency increased after the drug and insurance industries offered up their pledges to help with financing reform. Then the stakes increased further when the Obama Administration put out a proposal to cut payments to hospitals by $224 billion over the next ten years to help fund reform.[48]

A "preliminary agreement" was struck between the hospital industry, the White House and the Senate Finance Committee pledging that the industry would cut Medicare and Medicaid payments by $155 billion over ten years. Three organizations got together on this pledge: the Federation of American Hospitals (FAH, the trade group representing investor-owned hospitals), the Catholic Health Association (not-for-profit hospitals), and the American Hospital Association (AHA, representing all types of hospitals). The $155 billion pledge included projections to cut annual Medicare payments to hospitals ($103 billion), reducing re-admissions of patients to hospitals ($2 billion), and lowering federal Medicare and Medicaid payments to "disproportionate share" hospitals that provide care to uninsured and poor patients ($50 billion). The hospital organizations also expressed their cooperation with efforts to improve efficiencies and quality of care as well as testing ways to better integrate care, including the possibility of bundled payments.[49] The catch—this agreement was voluntary. It's hard to imagine that such cost savings—at the expense of hospitals—would have accrued simply because hospitals saw the wisdom of billing the government for less.

Once again, as we have seen with the insurance and drug industries, the hospital industry is sharply focused on preservation and growth of future revenue streams. While supporting expansion of insurance through the reform proposals, the industry expressed serious reservations about the public option and an independent commission with authority over Medicare spending.

One especially contentious issue, both within the hospital industry itself and in health policy circles, was the future role of so-called
specialty hospitals. These are physician-owned, for-profit facilities that
usually specialize in the care of insured patients needing procedures
in cardiovascular disease, orthopedic surgery and neurosurgery. They
have been criticized for cherry picking the market, not carrying their
share of emergency care (they seldom have emergency rooms), and
performing procedures even when unnecessary. They also involve "tri-
ple-dipping" by physicians who self-refer to their own facilities, then
receive income from doing the procedure, thereby sharing in the facil-
ity's profit and gaining in the value of their investment.[50]

The political battle over the future of specialty hospitals was
interesting to watch, and revealed whether reform could reduce
perverse incentives and cut costs in our market-based system. The
interests of specialty hospitals were being promoted by the San Diego-
based American Surgical Hospital Association, but were being opposed
by both the AHA and the FAH, which together represent most of the
hospitals in the country.[51] The Community Tracking Study carried
out by the Center for Studying Health System Change concluded that
"specialty hospitals are contributing to a medical arms race that is
driving up costs without demonstrating clear quality advantages."[52]

The initial House bill would have prevented the opening of new
specialty hospitals by disqualifying them from receiving payments from
Medicare, but would have grandfathered-in existing specialty hospitals.
Physician ownership would have been restricted to 40 percent. In
reaction, specialty hospitals began lobbying Congress heavily to restrict
such limits. For example, Doctors Hospital at Renaissance in Edinburg,
Texas, a 530- bed specialty hospital with physician ownership at the 82
percent level and with much higher levels of costs and utilization than
peer hospitals, raised at least $500,000 in a single fund-raising event for
the Democratic Senatorial Campaign Committee as well as more than
$800,000 for the Democratic Congressional Campaign Committee.[53]

Other tactics conducted by the hospital industry were generally in
favor of health care reform as it was developing, based on its expectation
that the large increase in the insured population would lead to increased
financial returns for hospitals. Not surprisingly, the FAH joined in a
$12 million advertising campaign by a new group called Americans for
Stable Quality Care, (which included such diverse coalition partners

as the AMA, Families USA, PhRMA and SEIU, the service employees' union), to support the goals of the Obama Administration.[54]

True to the pattern of other stakeholders, the hospital industry's $155 billion ten-year pledge to the reform effort would be more than offset by new revenues triggered by forcing every American to buy insurance. But as the individual mandate was progressively watered down in the Senate, the hospital industry became as wary as the insurance industry of their real costs of the reform bills.

The hospital industry became even more divided within itself, pitting lower-cost, more efficient hospitals in some more rural parts of the country against higher-cost urban hospitals in higher-spending regions, as well as general hospitals against physician and investor-owned specialty hospitals. Moreover, hospitals' interests deviated from other "allies", such as the medical device industry, over that industry's price-setting practices. Their typically confidential prices could vary, for example, from less than $2,000 for orthopedic hip components to more than $12,000 for the same product.[55]

As the bills made their way through Congress, the hospital industry had reason to fear for their future revenues. Researchers at Dartmouth Medical School's Institute for Health Policy and Clinical Research had estimated that up to one-third of all health care is either inappropriate or unnecessary, and that wide geographic disparities exist in the costs of medical care among Medicare patients in their last two years of life (e.g. $40,000 per patient at Genesis Medical Center in Davenport, Iowa vs. $105,000 per patient at New York University Langone Medical Center). The Dartmouth researchers further argued that Medicare spending could be cut by 15 to 30 percent without a drop in quality of care, and reduce the annual growth of per-patient spending from a national average of 3.5 percent to 2.4 percent, saving more than $1.42 trillion by 2023.[56] These kinds of studies would unquestionably work their way into future cuts in reimbursement for many hospitals, especially as legislators searched for ways to finance health care reform.

While continuing its overall support of the reform effort, especially with the prospect of up to 31 million new insured patients, the industry continued to lobby behind the scenes against cuts in Medicare reimbursement and other adverse impacts on its financial bottom line.

The final big player receiving health care dollars are physicians. Many if not most are staunch allies and advocates of their patients;

yet the AMA has for decades played a large role in thwarting reform efforts.

Organized Medicine: Show Me the Money

Since physicians order almost all services that are provided within our health care system, they are obviously a key player and interest group in the debate over health care reform.

Organized medicine has a poor track record in terms of reform. Although a universal system of health insurance was considered favorably for a short time by a committee of the American Medical Association (AMA) during Teddy Roosevelt's abortive attempt to establish such a program during the 1912 to 1917 period, the AMA has played a consistently reactionary role against such reform since then.

During the 1930s the AMA was a much stronger political force than it is today, to the extent that Franklin D. Roosevelt did not include national health insurance as part of his New Deal policies. Three decades later, the AMA fiercely opposed Medicare, branding it as socialized medicine and a government takeover.[57] It jumped on the bandwagon only after the American Hospital Association and Blue Cross got together in its support. Its initial opposition, however, soon turned to making best use of the program. Physicians' fees jumped almost eight percent in the first year after the program was enacted, more than twice the rise in the consumer price index.[58]

After World War II, organized medicine was fragmented into many smaller specialty and sub-specialty groups. As specialization advanced in following years, the AMA lost much of its political influence. Its membership dropped by 20 percent between 1993 and 2004.[59] The AMA represents less than one-quarter of the approximately 900,000 U.S. physicians, and the "house of medicine" is split into some 180 specialty and sub-specialty organizations and societies.

In the late spring of 2009, President Obama was busy getting the major stakeholders aboard his train for health care reform. We have seen how the insurance, drug and hospital industries made specific pledges in an effort to help pay for reform. While organized medicine made no such specific pledge, it was offered a deal by the White House if it would give its general support to the reform effort.

Once again, it was all about money. Whereas physicians had been facing cutbacks each year in Medicare reimbursement, usually reversed by Congress, the Obama Administration offered $245 billion to physicians as the "doc fix". At first, the Administration did not want to count this amount as costs of reform, but the CBO soon scored it as the additional costs that they are, coming up with a $239 billion increase in the federal deficit over the next ten years.[60]

So what were the attitudes among these many physician organizations toward the various reform proposals as they worked their way through Congress? True to form, the AMA and most groups were supportive of anything that would increase their reimbursement while opposing much else in the proposals. Reassured that the "doc fix" would provide more generous Medicare reimbursement (about 20 percent higher than it would have been under the original formula), at least for a time, the AMA and American College of Surgeons (ACS) expressed their support for the centerpiece of the reform bills—efforts to expand affordable health insurance through employer and individual mandates, subsidies for lower-income people to purchase insurance, and expansion of Medicaid. But for the AMA and most medical organizations, that is where their support melted away. Instead, they vigorously opposed these provisions:

- *The public option.* In a letter to the Senate Finance Committee, the AMA had this to say: "Creating a public health insurance option for non-disabled individuals under age 65 is not the best way to expand health insurance coverage and lower costs. The introduction of a new public plan threatens to restrict patient choice by driving out private insurers, which currently provide coverage for nearly 70 percent of Americans."[61]
- *An empowered independent Medicare rate-setting commission.* The AMA and ACS quickly expressed their opposition when White House budget director Peter Orszag proposed a new federal commission with the authority to set payment policy for physicians, hospitals, and other providers.[62]
- *Targeted Medicare reimbursement cuts.* In July 2009, the Administration proposed a plan to cut Medicare payments to cardiologists and oncologists by more than 10 percent each while increasing reimbursement to family physicians by 8 percent and nurses by 7 percent. This prompted leaders of the American College of Cardiology to warn: "The cuts could have the unintended consequences of rationing care, especially

in rural regions with a large number of Medicare patients. In other areas, specialists may decide to pull out of Medicare, or ask patients to make up the difference with higher out-of-pocket payments."[63]

Organized medicine has become so fragmented that no one group speaks for the profession. In fact, some groups have endorsed major health care reform, even to the point of single payer national health insurance (NHI). As the second largest medical organization in the country, with some 125,000 members, the American College of Physicians (ACP) has endorsed single payer as one of two major options to reform our system.[64] The American Public Health Association (APHA) has come out in favor of NHI. And of course, Physicians for a National Health Program (PNHP), a growing organization with 17,000 members, has pushed strongly for NHI since it was established in 1989. Meanwhile, many physicians across most specialties have come to see NHI as the only way to provide universal access to affordable health care. A large national survey involving more than 2,200 U.S. physicians in 2008 found that 59 percent supported government legislation to establish national health insurance.[65]

Most physicians do not see themselves as legitimate targets for cost containment measures, and want any increased reimbursement for primary care and other shortage fields to be an add-on rather than cuts in more highly reimbursed specialties. When a 5 percent tax on elective cosmetic surgery became part of the Senate bill (immediately dubbed the "Botax" after the anti-wrinkle product Botox), the American Academy of Cosmetic Surgery was quick to oppose it as a tax against women and the baby boomer generation.[66] The AMA spoke out against the tax as the first federal levy against a medical procedure.[67]

Physicians obviously had much to gain by reform bills that would convert tens of millions of uninsured to paying patients through one or another kind of mandated coverage. So their overall support of these bills was predictable. But most of their organizations continued to lobby against Medicare cuts, a Medicare Commission with rate-setting powers, the public option, and required reporting of physician performance data. Even after a study of more than 5,000 U.S. physicians found that 63 percent supported the public option and 58 percent supported expansion of Medicare to people 55 to 64 years of age,[68] the AMA continued to lobby against those changes. It gave its qualified support to H.R. 3962 only if the "doc fix" was also passed; after being voted down in the Senate, it became a new stand-alone House bill (H.R. 3961) with a $210 billion package for cancellation of the Sustainable Growth Rate Formula reimbursement cuts.

THE CORPORATE "ALLIANCE": SERVING THEMSELVES OR THE PUBLIC?

Having considered the voluntary, unenforceable pledges, together with the agendas and subsequent actions by five of the major stakeholders, it is now useful to reassess the impacts on reform by the corporate "alliance" struck at that time. Table 1.3 summarizes the pledges, agendas, tactics and likely rewards for the Big Four stakeholders.

As is evident from Table 1.3, all four stakeholders would have done well with health care reform along the lines of bills then before Congress. The House bill (H.R. 3200), with a cost of some $1 trillion over 10 years and without effective cost containment mechanisms, would have added greatly to the revenues of all corporate stakeholders in the medical industrial complex. Their revenues, however, are *our* costs, especially since the insurance industry will likely be protected by lenient standards (such as a requirement that insurance cover only 60 to 70 percent of health care costs).

The Big Four that we have looked at are only part of the cost problem. There are many other major players in the health care industry, mostly investor-owned, with a primary mission to make money, not save the money of patients, their families and taxpayers. These players range from medical device and equipment industries to nursing homes and health information technology companies. For example, General Electric, the 12th largest corporation in the world, has a big market share for imaging equipment and information technology. While GE initiated a major national advertising campaign supporting health care reform, its lobbyists were fighting against cuts in Medicare reimbursement for imaging procedures.[69] The 3,300 lobbyists then in Washington, D.C. were spending $1.4 million dollars a day lobbying for one or another health care interest, for or against specific provisions in the proposals before Congress

Most health care industries welcome government subsidies to grow the insured population, but not at the price of burdensome regulation. There is little common ground among the stakeholders in the medical industrial complex except the goal to expand markets and grow

TABLE 1.3

CORPORATE "ALLIANCE" FOR HEALTH CARE REFORM - THE BIG FOUR

Insurance Industry

Pledge	Abandon pre-existing conditions as an underwriting principle
	Accept all applicants
	Stop charging women higher premiums than men
Agenda	Grow private and public insurance markets by up to 50 million enrollees
Tactics	Oppose controls or caps on premium rates
	Oppose the public option
	Lobby for low standards for insurance coverage and low MLRs
	Fight against cuts of overpayments for Medicare Advantage plans
Rewards	Larger private and public markets
	Higher profits and returns to shareholders
	Preempt increased regulation by government

PhRMA

Pledge	$80 billion over 10 years toward costs of health care reform
Agenda	Expand private and public markets
	Avoid price controls and competition from importation of drugs from other countries
	Gain maximal patent protection for biotech drugs
Tactics	With assurance from White House agreement that government would not negotiate drug prices or import drugs from abroad, lobbied jointly with Families USA in support of health care reform as represented by bills in Congress
Rewards	Expanded private and public markets
	Higher profits and returns to shareholders
	Avoid increased regulation by government

Hospital Industry

Pledge	$155 billion over 10 years in reduced hospital charges
Agenda	Growth in future revenues in private and public markets
Tactics	Lobby for employer and individual mandates, and expansion of Medicaid
Rewards	Larger private and public markets
	Increased revenues ($170 billion), more than offsetting its pledged amount (40)

Organized Medicine

Pledge	No specific pledge
Agenda	Support private markets and restrain government intervention
	Prevent cuts in Medicare reimbursement
Tactics	Supports employer and individual mandates, insurance reforms, and expansion of Medicaid
	Opposes public option, rate-setting by independent commission, and targeted reimbursement cuts by specialty
Rewards	$245 billion "doc fix" restores Medicare reimbursement, at least for a time
	Increased revenues from expanded insured population

future profits for each industry. The "alliance" is in name only, hardly partners in most instances. When their respective interests conflict with other corporate stakeholders, the circular firing squad starts shooting. Examples include the insurance trade group AHIP's battle against physicians' high out-of-network fees, while medical organizations sue insurers for non-payment of fees and call for elimination of overpayments to private Medicare plans.

As the battles raged on between and among corporate stakeholders, their lobbyists, and reformers in and out of government, the public interest was being overlooked as stakeholders worked toward carving out a bigger piece of an expanded revenue pie for themselves. The neutering of the public option was but one of many examples whereby the public was losing out. Instead of cost-containment in a reform bill, we could expect to see continued inflation of health care costs at rates much higher than cost-of-living or median wages. Judging from the bills taking shape in Congress, the likely outcome would be a bonanza for health care industries and a bailout for an unaffordable and dying insurance industry.

By the time of the Congressional recess in August, Bob Herbert, well-known Op-Ed columnist for the *New York Times*, was right on target with this observation:

> "The drug companies, the insurance industry and the rest of the corporate high-rollers have their tentacles all over this so-called reform effort, squeezing it for all it's worth. Meanwhile, the public—struggling with the worst economic downturn since the 1930s—is looking on with great anxiety and confusion. If the drug companies and the insurance industry are smiling, it can only mean that the public interest is being left behind."[70]

Wrapped in language of cooperation and a shared goal of improving the health care system, Obama's summit and his rhetoric concealed a basic truth: reform was unlikely to work because of the disparate agendas, and if it did come to pass, it would only do so at the expense of the very people it was purportedly trying to help: the public. The only way these parties could embrace change would be if it were a win for their investors—that's how the system works. Thus these companies can only be made to embrace change, to make them advocates of change, when that change runs counter to the goals of real health care reform: efficient delivery of medical care that is accessible to all. Under these consensus-building reform attempts, universal access is possible—if it allows for inefficient delivery that the public is forced to pay for.

The End Result: A Circular Firing Squad over Prices and Costs

Among these major corporate stakeholders of U.S. health care, all are quick to point fingers at others for causing the continued soaring costs of care. Each has its own defense for why it is not their fault. Insurers say that hospitals, drug companies and physicians are overcharging them, leaving them no choice but to raise premiums. Hospitals point to the increasing clout of physicians to demand higher payments, as well as their rising burden of care for the uninsured and low reimbursement from Medicare and Medicaid. Drug companies say they need their prices to continue to innovate new drugs, although many studies show that few new drugs are improvements over older drugs, that Europe with lower prices brings more breakthroughs to market than the U.S., and that the industry spends two and a half times as much on marketing and advertising than on R&D.[71]

Each of the stakeholders is right to an extent—*but they all contribute to the cost problem*. And the power dynamics among them are constantly changing. Robert Laszewski, president of the consulting firm Health Policy & Strategy Associates, has this to say:

> "It's always someone else's fault. There is not an incentive for these people to cooperate because the game they are playing is getting a bigger piece of the pie."[72]

As an example in northern California, Sutter Health owns two dozen hospitals and medical centers, and Catholic Healthcare West runs 33 hospitals. With their negotiating clout, they are now commanding annual double-digit payment increases. Angela Braly, Wellpoint's CEO, says that dominant hospital systems are demanding 40 percent rate increases while drug companies seek 20 percent profit margins.[73] On the basis of these kinds of cost increases, researchers at the Center for Studying Health System Change are now predicting that proposed accountable care organizations (ACOs) may be ineffective in moderating costs and may actually lead to higher rates for private payers.[74]

Beyond casting blame for health care inflation on other stakeholders, they are becoming more confrontational with each other. A good example is the bitter contract dispute playing out between Continuum Health Partners, a consortium of five New York hospitals, and UnitedHealthcare. The battle is over rates as well as UnitedHealth's demand that hospitals notify the insurer within 24 hours of a patient's admission to the hospital—failure to do so would result in a cut in hospital reimbursement by one-half.[75]

But the political wars were just starting over health care reform. In the next chapters, we will examine other forces lining up against health care reform in the public interest—the forces we will continue to be up against in the ongoing fight for single payer.

References

1. Obama, B. Transcript: Obama's acceptance speech. Election night, Chicago, IL, *Yahoo News*. November 4, 2008.
2. Machiavelli, N. *Brainy Quote.*
3. Peterson, MA. Political influence in the 1990s: From iron triangles to policy networks. *J Health Polit Policy Law* 18 (2):395-438, 1993.
4. Pear, R. Health care's early pledges. *New York Times*, May 12, 2009: A1.
5. Koffler, K. The Rose Garden: Administration exaggerates alliances on reform. *Roll Call*, July 27, 2009.
6. Meckler, L, Fuhrmans, V. Insurers offer to end prices tied to illness. *Wall Street Journal*, March 25, 2009: A4.
7. Kaiser Daily Health Policy Report, May 28, 2009.
8. Terhune, C, Epstein, K. Why health insurers are winning. *BusinessWeek*. August 17, 2009: 036.
9. Britt, R. WellPoint faces firestorm over hikes, profits. *Market Watch*, February 10, 2010.
10. Yee, CM. UnitedHealth profit soars 155%. *Star Tribune*, July 21, 2009.
11. Murphy, T. Insurer UnitedHealth sharply raises dividend. Associated Press, May 26, 2010.
12. Ibid #8.
13. Tracy, T. UnitedHealth, Aetna, WellPoint get bullish signal. *Wall Street Journal*, August 18, 2009: C3.
14. Johnson, A. Insurers tally up Baucus bill provisions. *Wall Street Journal*, September 28, 2009: A4.
15. Abelson, R. Senate pressing insurers on the amount of premiums they spend on care. *New York Times*, November 3, 2009: B1.
16. Hitt, G, Adamy, J. Insurers push back as Senate health vote nears. *Wall Street Journal*, October 13, 2009: A4.
17. Sack, K. Dealing with being the health care 'villains'. *New York Times*, August 28, 2009: A12.

18. Beebe, P. Regence campaign: Consumers must make choices to reduce health care costs. *Salt Lake Tribune*, October 14, 2009.

19. Pear, R, Herszenhorn, DM. White House and Democrats call insurance industry report on premiums flawed. *New York Times*, October 13, 2009: A13.

20. Feder, JL. Crafting health reform. *The Nation* 289 (15), November 9, 2009, pp 4-5.

21. Eggen, D. Insurer enlists employees to fight health reform. *Washington Post*, November 13, 2009.

22. Appleby, J, Carey, MA. Democrats' ideas to expand Medicare raise hackles of doctors, hospitals, insurers. *Kaiser Health News*, December 9, 2009.

23. Abelson, R. In battle's aftermath, for most, big changes are not expected. *New York Times*, December 25, 2009: A1.

24. Stone, P. Health insurers funded Chamber attack ads. *National Journal*, January 12, 2010.

25. Johnson, A. Fight over health-care premiums heats up. *Wall Street Journal*, February 19, 2010: A6.

26. Seelye, KQ. Administration rejects health insurer's defense of huge rate increases. *New York Times*, February 12, 2010: A17.

27. Johnson, LA. Anthem to delay insurance rate hike amid criticism. Associated Press. February 14, 2010.

28. Gonzales, J. Insurance premium hikes hit small business hard. San Francisco Chronicle, June 12, 2010.

29. Press release. California Nurses Association. RNs praise Atty Gen. move to subpoena insurance plans, Move follows nurses report on patient claims data denials—*NEW DATA*—Denial rates averaged 26 percent even after public uproar. Sacramento, CA, February 25, 2010.

30. U.S. House of Representatives, Committee on Energy and Commerce. Washington, D.C., February 24, 2010.

31. Lueck, S. Tauzin is named top lobbyist for pharmaceutical industry, *Wall Street Journal*, December 16, 2004: A4.

32. Pear, R. Federal saving in drug price cut unclear. *New York Times*, June 23, 2009: A15.

33. Grim, R. Internal memo confirms big giveaways in White House deal with big PhRMA. *Huffington Post*, August 13, 2009.

34. Kirkpatrick, DD. House leaders say no to cost cap for drug makers. *New York Times*, August 7, 2009: A11.

35. Singer, N. Harry and Louise return, with a new message. *New York Times*, July 17, 2009: B3.

36. Rovner, J. Opponents support expanding Medicaid coverage. *NPR*, April 20, 2009.

37. Richwine, L. Senate panel backs 12-year biotech drug shelter. *Reuters*, July 13, 2009.

38. Mundy, A, Meckler, L. Drug makers score early. *Wall Street Journal*, July 17, 2009: A2.

39. Adamy, J, Hitt, G. CEOs tally health-bill score. *Wall Street Journal*, October 19, 2009: A3.

40. Murray, M. PhRMA-funded ads tout health care reform. *Roll Call*, November 23, 2009.
41. Kirkpatrick, DD. Groups back overhaul, but seek cover. *New York Times*, September 12, 2009: A1.
42. Harris, G. Drug makers are advocacy group's biggest donors. *New York Times*, October 22, 2009: A25.
43. Wilson, D. Drug companies increase prices in face of change. *New York Times*, November 16, 2009: A1.
44. Kirkpatrick, DD. Drug industry girds for rise in its share of overhaul. *New York Times*, December 23, 2009: A16.
45. Kirkpatrick, DD. At state level, health lobby fights change. *New York Times*, December 29, 2009.
46. Kirkpatrick, DD, Wilson, D. One grand deal too many costs Tauzin his job. *New York Times*, February 13, 2010: B1.
47. Galewitz, P. Checking in with Chip Kahn: 'Potential for hospitals and our patients to be big winners.' *Kaiser Daily News*, August 23, 2009.
48. Adamy, J, Rockoff, JD. Hospital industry bristles at cuts. *Wall Street Journal*, June 15, 2009: A3.
49. Medicare Rights Center. White House announces deal with hospitals to cut Medicare and Medicaid payments. *Medicare Watch*, issue 14, July 15, 2009.
50. Medicare Payment Advisory Commission. *Report to the Congress: Physician-Owned Specialty Hospitals*. Washington D.C.: MedPAC, March 8, 2005.
51. Szabo, J. Washington Watch. Medicare law bans some doctor-owned hospitals. *Physicians Financial News* 22:2, February 15, 2005, p 13.
52. Berenson, RA, Bazzoli, FGJ, Au, M. Do specialty hospitals promote price competition? Center for Studying Health System Change. Issue Brief No. 103, January, 2006.
53. Sack, K, Herszenhorn, DM. Texas hospital flexing its muscle in health fight. *New York Times*, July 30, 2009: A1.
54. Kaiser Daily Health Policy Report, August 13, 2009, *Kaiser Health News*, p 6.
55. Kamp, J. Hospitals face price uncertainty on devices. *Wall Street Journal*, November 4, 2009: B7.
56. Hartocollis, A. Hospitals cite worry on fees in health bill. *New York Times*, November 3, 2009: A1.
57. Marmor, TR. *The Politics of Medicare*. New York. Aldine Publishing Company, 1970, pp 27-31.
58. Ibid #57.
59. *Chicago Tribune.* American Medical Association overhauls its image in new marketing effort. Posted June 17, 2005
60. Adamy, J. Doctors' payments snag health bill. *Wall Street Journal*, July 20, 2009: A3.
61. Pear, R. Doctors' group opposes public health insurance plan. *New York Times,* June 11, 2009: A17.
62. Goldstein, J. Doctors oppose giving commission power over Medicare payments. *Wall Street Journal*, July 29, 2009: A3.
63. Nussbaum, A, Rapaport, L. Cardiologists crying foul over Obama Medicare

cuts (Update 1). *Bloomberg News*, August 28, 2009.

64. American College of Physicians. Position Paper. *Achieving a High Performance Health Care System with Universal Access: What the United States Can Learn from Other Countries. Ann Intern Med*, January 1, 2008.

65. Carroll, AE, Ackermann, RT. Support for national health insurance among U.S. physicians: Five years later. *Ann Intern Med* 148: 566-7, 2008.

66. Galewitz, P. Plastic surgeons cry foul over 'Botax' proposal in Senate health bill. *Kaiser Health News*, November 20, 2009.

67. Rockoff, JD. Knives drawn over 'Botax'. *Wall Street Journal*, December 4, 2009: A3.

68. Keyhani, S, Federman, A. Doctors on coverage—Physicians' views on a new public insurance option and Medicare expansion. *New Engl J Med* 361(14): October 1, 2009.

69. Adamy, J, Williamson, E. As Congress goes on break, health lobbying heats up. *Wall Street Journal*, August 5, 2009: A1.

70. Herbert, B. This is reform? *New York Times*, August 17, 2009.

71. Light, DW. Global drug discovery: Europe is ahead. *Health Affairs Web Exclusive* W969. August 25, 2009.

72. Johnson, A. Race to pin blame for health costs. *Wall Street Journal*, February 26, 2010: A5.

73. Ibid #72.

74. Berenson, RA, Ginsburg, PB, Kemper, N. Unchecked provider clout in California foreshadow challenges to health reform. *Health Affairs* online, February 25, 2010.

75. Hartocollis, A. Insurer steps up fight to control health care cost. *New York Times*, January 24, 2010.

CHAPTER 2

Corruption of the Political Process: How Industry Shepherds its Legislators

"There are two important things in politics. The first is the money and I can't remember the second."
— Mark Hanna, campaign manager
to President William McKinley

"It is a truism in the political economy of the U.S. health care sector that costs are so difficult to control because every dollar in cost savings is a dollar less income for one or more interest groups. Health reform will necessarily be redistributive. As the health reform debate heats up in the coming months and years, the likely losers from such a redistribution will seek to deflect the discussion to blaming patients, government, or each other as the source of cost problems. We would all be better served, we believe, if the issues of who wins and who loses were made more open and explicit."
— Bruce Vladeck, former administrator, Health Care Financing
Administration, now CMS, and Thomas Rice, Professor of Health Services,
UCLA School of Public Health[1]

Stakeholders in our profit-making, largely investor-owned market-based health care system have an entrenched and sophisticated system, lubricated by generous transfers of money, influencing policymakers, burnishing their image and persuading the public that they are all on the same side.

What kind of political muscle do those of us favoring single payer need to develop to win? The reform efforts of 2009-2010 did a great deal to obscure just who wins and who loses in the health care battle, and how powerful they are. Even as President Obama lashed out against insurance companies, it was pretty clear they would be among the winners in his solution. It was left to Republicans and a few progressives to point out who loses in a market people are forced to join: the American public. We need a clear-eyed view of who would lose— and the extent to which they will keep fighting to corrupt our political will and our democratic institutions.

In this chapter we size up the raw financial and political power faced by those of us who want real change. We will look more closely at: (1) ways in which industry courts legislators and policymakers to do their bidding, and (2) how corporate power continues to undermine the public interest.

SAUSAGE FOR SALE: DINNER ON K STREET

These are some of the major ways by which corporate interests purchase goodwill with policymakers and legislators and help to shape legislation involving health care.

Lobbyists

Lobbyists descended on our nation's capitol like locusts when Congress began debating health care reform. Bill Allison, a senior fellow at the Sunshine Foundation, a Washington D.C.-based watchdog group, observed:

> "When you have a big piece of legislation like this, it's like ringing the dinner bell for K Street... There's a lot of money at stake and there are a lot of special interests who don't want their ox gored."[2]

By mid-August 2009, 3,300 lobbyists representing more than 1,500 organizations were at work on the health care issue alone (three times the number of defense lobbyists), with three more joining up every day. Over a full range of issues, there were more than 12,000 federally registered lobbyists in Washington D.C. But that number grossly understates the army of people involved in the political advocacy business. James Thurber, director of the Center for Congressional and Presidential Studies at American University, estimated that 90,000 to 120,000 unregistered people were working in one or another capacity in political advocacy, whether as astroturfers, strategists, or in other ways. By his count, there were about 168 influence peddlers for every member of Congress.[3]

A February 2010 analysis of Senate lobbying disclosure forms by the Center for Public Integrity found that more than 1,750 companies and organizations hired about 4,525 lobbyists—eight for each member of Congress—to influence health care legislation in 2009. These included 207 hospitals, 105 insurance companies, 85 manufacturing companies and 745 trade, advocacy and professional organizations. According to the non-profit Center for Responsive Politics, 2009 was a record year for influence peddling overall with business and advocacy groups spending $3.47 billion on lobbyists.[4]

Spending on lobbying by the health care sector skyrocketed in the 1998 to 2008 period, as shown by Figure 2.1. In the second quarter of 2009, health care players spent $133 million promoting their interests, according to the non-partisan Center for Responsive Politics. And many other interests joined in the lobbying frenzy, from labor unions to the U.S. Chamber of Commerce. This became a feeding frenzy over

FIGURE 2.1

Spending by Health Care Industry on Lobbying, 1998-2009

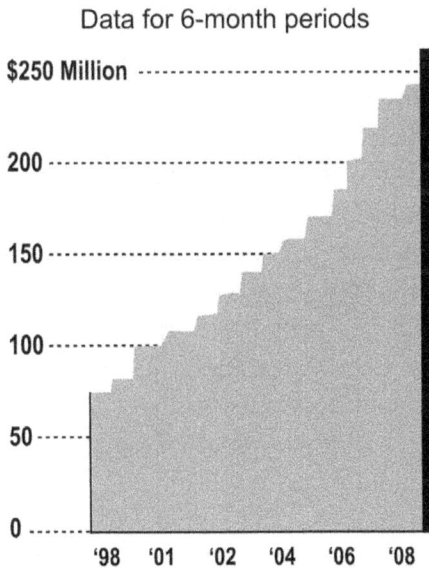

Data for 6-month periods

Source: Center for Responsive Politics. Reprinted with permission from Adamy, J, Williamson, E. As Congress goes on break, health lobbying heats up. *Wall Street Journal*, August 5, 2009: A1.

getting a bigger piece of the future revenue pie from whatever bill finally emerged from Congress. Some lobbyists were blunt in admitting
that their interest was not in cost containment, but rather protecting and
growing their future markets. For example, Tim Trysla, executive director of the Access to Medical Imaging Coalition, lobbied 120 legislators, sometimes together with General Electric representatives, arguing
against cuts in reimbursement for such imaging procedures as CT and
MRI scans. In his words: "If you're looking for savings, don't come at
us."[5]

Lobbyists concerned with health care legislation come at it from
all angles, often dividing longtime allies whenever their particular revenue streams may be threatened. These examples suggest how diverse
these issues are and how high the potential stakes are for respective
interests:

- Lobbyists for Genentech, a large biotechnology manufacturer
  of specialty cancer drugs, carried out a lobbying blitz targeting
  Congressional staff members of both parties in an effort to
  secure as many supportive statements "as humanly possible" to
  raise the patent protection from generic drugs by an additional
  12 years; it was estimated that 22 Republicans and 20 Democrats
  picked up the talking points, which then became verbatim parts
  of the Congressional Record.[6]
- The Community Oncology Alliance, which spent $200,000
  on lobbyists in the second quarter of 2009, brought 100
  oncologists to Capitol Hill in July to demand that proposed cuts
  in reimbursement under Medicare for cancer drugs be reversed.
  Oncologists commonly receive lucrative kickbacks from drug
  companies for administering these drugs, and lobbied to continue
  these reimbursement arrangements as part of their increasing
  costs.[7] But this is an important cause of soaring costs—the costs
  of cancer care are rising by about 20 percent a year, and cancer
  drugs are leading the surge in these costs.[8]
- Deviating from many other business interests, Wal-Mart
  supported an employer mandate. The giant discount retailer had
  been widely known as a miserly employer for health benefits
  with much of its workforce uninsured or underinsured. Wal-Mart
  came under immediate fire from the National Retail Federation,

the industry's biggest trade group, for its backing of the employer mandate. The industry is plagued by high turnover rates of lower-income employees. Less than one-half of retailers offer their workers any health insurance, and typically that involves high deductibles and minimal benefits. Other retailers saw Wal-Mart's endorsement of an employer mandate as a shrewd PR effort to improve its reputation when it was becoming clear that an employer mandate would be part of health care legislation.[9]

- The Mayer Brown law firm was paid more than $110,000 in 2009 to lobby for requiring insurers to consider covering Christian Science prayer treatments under health care bills in Congress.[10]

Health care industries targeted both political parties in their lobbying effort, with special focus on those best placed to shape health reform bills, especially members of the Senate Finance Committee. Appointment books of many legislators were filled with lobbyists of many stripes. As reported on NPR's *All Things Considered,* Senate Finance Committee Chairman Max Baucus rotated weekly meetings among various groups—providers one week, purchasers a second, consumers a third. The Sunlight Foundation made a map of the Baucus Health Care Lobbyist Complex.[11] As Larry McNeely, a health care advocate with the Boston-based U.S. Public Interest Research Group, said: "The sheer quantity of money that's sloshed around Washington is drowning out the voices of citizens and the groups that speak up for them."[12]

From industry perspectives, this was money well spent, blocking such provisions as the public option and other cost-cutting measures. The 33 lobbyists deployed by the AMA helped kill a tax on cosmetic surgery, cuts in Medicare payments to primary care physicians, and a $300 yearly fee for physicians who participate in Medicare or Medicaid. As Julian Zelizer, Professor of Public Affairs at Princeton University, observed about this entire lobbying campaign:

> "They cut it. They chopped it. They reconstructed it. They didn't bury it. I don't think they wanted to."[13]

Beyond the hordes of registered lobbyists, there was another large group of *unregistered* lobbyists. In her recent book, *The Shadow Elite: How the World's New Power Brokers Undermine Democracy,*

Government, and the Free Market, Janine Wedel, Professor of Public Policy and Social Anthropology at George Mason University, sheds light on this underground world of influence peddling.[14] Tom Daschle, former Democratic Senator from South Dakota and Senate Majority Leader, is a good example of this group. Despite efforts by Congress to tighten lobbyist regulations over the past two years, a loophole allows lobbyists to bypass registration if they spend less than 20 percent of their time on lobbying. Daschle makes use of this loophole as he advises colleagues and private clients on health care policy as a member of the lobbying firm, Alston and Bird.[15]

There is another variant of the lobbyist role that further extends the reach of corporate cash on political decision-making—the "political intelligence" industry. The oldest political intelligence firm in Washington, D.C. is Washington Analysis Corp., started in the early 1970s by Les Alperstein, its current president. Today there are many competing firms in this growing industry. These firms employ experts on health care, financial services, energy and other areas who are recruited from Capitol Hill offices and even some media outlets to closely track economic policy, legislation and regulations. They can alert their employers and clients to worrisome developments within minutes. One recent example occurred late on the morning of January 6, 2010, when a rumor flew through the Capitol that Congressional Democrats were considering imposing a $750 million annual fee on clinical laboratories as a way of helping to pay for the health care reform bill. After some frantic calls to House and Senate aides, the rumor was found to be untrue, but not before the stocks of Quest Diagnostics, Genoptix and Laboratory Corp. all fell sharply. The political intelligence operatives work in the shadows, and are not subject to the same disclosure requirements as lobbyists are.[16]

Campaign Contributions and Political Action Committees (PACs)

Eric Cantor, Republican Congressman from Virginia, has a PAC called ERIC (Every Republican Is Crucial). In July, ERIC rented a 15,000 square foot party space at Nationals Park, a major league baseball stadium, for the "Cantor Festival". It was a private affair. The "requested contribution" was $5,000. Guests could take batting practice, play video games at the Sony PlayStation "pavilion", and listen to the band Blame It On Jane, which performed at the Republican National

Convention. From the large sums raised (ERIC collected $119,000 in July alone, but much of these contributions go unreported), Cantor gave away almost one-half to fellow legislators. As a result, he was elected the minority whip, the second-ranking Republican in the House. Many of the "hosts" for events like this are also lobbyists. In this case, they included representatives from the American College of Surgeons as well as the drug and medical device industries. As a member of the House Ways and Means Committee, Cantor has legislative jurisdiction over health care, Medicare and prescription drugs for seniors. In addition to events like this, Cantor is readily available for a "chat" at a Washington D.C. Starbucks—at a cost of $2,500 per PAC.[17]

By the spring of 2009, it became clear that the Senate Finance Committee would play a key role in deciding what kinds of health care reform, if any, would be passed by Congress. Its 23 members included 13 Democrats and 10 Republicans. They have all benefited for years from the largesse of special interest PACs related to health care, including the AMA, the AHA, PhRMA, medical device and insurance companies. Table 2.1 lists contributions from the health sector, as well as the insurance industry, to these 23 legislators for 2008 and over their careers.[18]

As the health care debate wound on, it also became clear that Blue Dog Democrats, centrist fiscal conservatives with mounting concerns over proposed health care bills, would also play pivotal roles in brokering outcomes of reform legislation. The 52 members of the Blue Dog Coalition set a record pace for fundraising through its PAC, raising more than $1.1 million over the first six months of 2009.[19]

Health care industries targeted key politicians of both parties and in both chambers of Congress. Industry bought off many members of Congress, on both sides of the aisle, and multiplied its efforts by concentrating on legislators most pivotal to the content of bills working their way through Congress. The political impact of just 13 legislators in both parties in two key committees in Congress—the Senate Finance Committee and the House Energy and Commerce Committee—was playing a big role in determining the outcome of any bill that might emerge. They come from small states and rural areas, and together represent only 13 million people, just 4 percent of the population upon whom they are imposing their views on health care. By the summer of 2009, these 13 lawmakers had already raised $12 million for their campaigns.[20]

TABLE 2.1

Contributions to Democratic Senators

SENATOR	2008 HEALTH SECTOR	CAREER HEALTH SECTOR	2008 INSURANCE SECTOR	CAREER INSURANCE SECTOR
Max Baucus (MT)	$1,148,775	$2,797,381	$285,850	$1,170,313
John D. Rockefeller IV (WV)	$515,150	$1,674,229	$107,874	$394,074
Kent Conrad (ND)	$117,350	$1,331,363	$56,650	$821,187
Jeff Bingaman (NM)	$14,151	$861,841	$1,500	$160,875
John F. Kerry (MA)	$289,430	$8,145,141	$90,250	$1,397,367
Blanche L. Lincoln (AR)	$226,753	$1,281,608	$49,500	$440,033
Ron Wyden (OR)	$96,925	$1,161,488	$45,999	$229,173
Charles E. Schumer (NY)	$10,000	$1,402,358	$3,000	$946,400
Debbie Stabenow (MI)	$239,018	$1,118,186	$40,800	$246,750
Maria Cantwell (WA)	$48,951	$573,076	$12,300	$80,850
Bill Nelson (FL)	$60,015	$1,163,210	$22,500	$520,016
Robert Menendez (NJ)	$81,650	$1,216,476	$67,450	$458,679
Thomas Carper (DE)	$15,450	$452,000	$28,700	$447,984

Source: Center for Responsive Politics. Editorial. Puppets in Congress. *New York Times*, November 17, 2009:A28.

TABLE 2.1 (continued)

Contributions to Republican Members of the Senate Finance Committee

SENATOR	2008 HEALTH SECTOR	CAREER HEALTH SECTOR	2008 INSURANCE SECTOR	CAREER INSURANCE SECTOR
Chuck Grassley (IA)	$334,237	$1,876,479	$72,200	$858,224
Orrin G. Hatch (UT)	$122,300	$2,311,744	$24,880	$659,307
Olympia J. Snowe (ME)	$6,000	$744,640	$5,000	$408,490
Jon Kyl (AZ)	$68,550	$1,971,968	$2,000	$533,044
Jim Bunning (KY)	$40,450	$1,045,687	$45,100	$769,016
Mike Crapo (ID)	$92,000	$549,192	$63,750	$360,932
Pat Roberts (KS)	$657,749	$903,337	$157,900	$296,342
John Ensign (NV)	$16,550	$1,795,899	$19,150	$580,690
Mike Enzil (WY)	$287,549	$612,715	$84,250	$240,953
John Cornyn (TX)	$950,669	$1,994,353	$289,069	$568,253

Source: Center for Responsive Politics. Editorial. Puppets in Congress. *New York Times*, November 17, 2009:A28.

As each Blue Dog Democrat raised concerns over particular provisions in health care bills making their way through Congress, industry benefactors were quick to fill their campaign coffers. Michael Ross (D-AR), a Blue Dog leader against the public option, received nearly $1 million in contributions from the health care sector and insurance industry over his five terms in Congress.[21] He parroted the insurance industry's claim that a government-run public plan would reduce competition and drive insurers out of business.[22] Insurers recognize they cannot compete against a not-for-profit public plan with low administrative costs.[23]

According to the Center for Responsive Politics, the health care industry contributed $20.5 million to federal legislators and the political parties during the first six months of 2009. Senate Majority Leader Harry Reid led the parade, garnering $382,400 toward his 2010 re-election campaign.[24] The health insurance industry did its part to ensure political attention to its interests. Table 2.2 lists the contributions by three large insurers and AHIP, their national trade group, from 2005 to 2008. These contributions were directed to legislators in both parties who were in pivotal positions to shape or scuttle specific provisions in health reform bills.[25] By October 2009, legislators up for election in 2010 had received $23 million in their campaign war chests.[26]

As the second largest insurer in the country, UnitedHealth put on a road show in July with a promotional bus displaying a sign declaring *Connecting You to a World of Care.* Across the country, Democrat after Democrat climbed aboard as the company burnished its image as supportive of health care reform. Judah Sommer, head of UnitedHealth's Washington D.C. office, offered: "This puts a halo on us. It humanizes us. "[27]

Revolving Doors for Influence Peddling

Elizabeth Fowler is the chief health advisor for Senator Max Baucus, chairman of the influential Senate Finance Committee. *Politico* has tagged her as the "chief operating officer" for the health care reform process. But she is really an insurance industry insider, having served as vice president of public policy for WellPoint, the country's largest insurer, from 2006 to 2008. She is widely recognized as the lead author of the Senate Finance Committee bill. When she was appointed to her current job, Baucus praised her for her expertise in health policy, and

TABLE 2.2

Insuring Political Attention
Campaign Contributions by These Major Health Carriers
Illustrate One Way They Seek Influence in Washington

INSURER	2005-2006	2007-2008
Blue Cross/Blue Shield	$2,451,716	$3,125,921
AFLAC	$1,924,335	$2,211,030
UnitedHealth Group	$1,045,877	$1,568,634
Aetna	$674,950	$721,957
America's Health Insurance Plans	$510,561	$591,750

Source: Cummings, J. When D.C. rumors move markets. Politico, January 19, 2010.

the media failed to report her ties to industry. Before Fowler, Baucus' chief health advisor was Michelle Easton, who moved on to lobby for WellPoint as a principal at the large lobbying firm Tarplin, Downs & Young.[28]

Other staff members for the Senate Finance Committee's "Gang of Six" have been back and forth through the revolving door with the insurance industry. Stephen Northrup was the former chief health advisor for Senator Mike Enzi (R-WY) from 2003 to 2006. He had a hand in writing provisions of a bill introduced by Enzi in 2006 that would allow insurers to be accountable only to the state with the most lenient regulatory requirements. In 2007 he joined WellPoint as vice president of federal affairs in Washington, D.C. According to *Modern Healthcare*, he is "responsible for leading WellPoint's advocacy efforts before Congress and various federal government agencies." This was not Northrup's first time through the revolving door—after serving as director of the Long Term Care Pharmacy Alliance, he had joined Enzi's staff to help craft the 2003 Medicare legislation that created the Part D prescription drug plan, which has been a bonanza for the drug industry.[29]

So in effect, WellPoint had a strong hand, if not the main hand, in writing the Senate Finance Committee's bill. That bill killed the public option, meeting the goal of Northrup and his employer. This is how Bill Moyers and Michael Winship of the weekly *Bill Moyers Journal* on PBS summed up the insurance industry's campaign to kill the public option:

> "They want a public option about as much as you want the swine flu, and just to be certain Congress sticks with the program, the industry has been showering megabucks all over Capitol Hill. From the beginning, they wanted to make sure that whatever bill comes out of the Finance Committee puts for-profit insurance companies first – by forcing the uninsured to buy medical policies from them. Money not only talks, it writes the prescriptions."[30]

One of those eager to fill the prescriptions was Richard Gephardt. Though he often voted with establishment interests over some 28 years in national Democratic politics, he promoted himself as a populist champion for ordinary Americans, including support for universal health care. As a presidential candidate in 2003, he condemned corporate crime as "ruining people's lives for selfishness and greed." Leaving office in 2005, he turned to lobbying, and before long formed his own lobbying firm, the Gephardt Group. In his new role, his earlier principles vanished. He became especially active in advising the insurance and drug industries. He helped UnitedHealth in its battle against the public option. He lobbied directly for PhRMA, even calling at one time for a federal "bailout of the pharmaceutical industry." He has a large lobbying contract with The Medicines Company, which focuses on drugs for critical care patients, and chairs the Council for American Medical Innovation (CAMI), which was formed by PhRMA. CAMI's agenda is to extend patents and block cheaper generic drugs from the market. The Gephardt Group brought in more than $2.4 million in the first half of 2009, a 50 percent jump over the first half of 2008 (an understated figure since other income by unregistered advocates went unreported). As Sebastian Jones wrote in a 2009 issue of *The Nation*:

> "Taken as a whole, Gephardt's success represents two distinct problems. For Democrats, it raises the legitimate question of whether his ideological shift from progressive populist to big

business champion is indicative of where the entire party is headed after two successive electoral victories. For Washington, it exposes the rot at the core and the insidious manner in which Gephardt has harnessed his media-anointed, colleague-respected role as an expert on issues of labor and universal healthcare to work against reforms for both."[31]

These are not isolated examples, but more the rule than the exception. According to the Medill News Service, a program of Northwestern University's Medill School of Journalism, and the Center for Responsive Politics, by late 2009 there were at least 166 former aides from nine congressional leadership offices and five committees involved in health care legislation working as health care lobbyists, together with 13 former legislators, all with salaries much higher than members of Congress.[32]

"Information Feeds" from Industry to Legislators

Public relations and research arms of industry are ready and willing to prepare reports on issues within the purview of selected legislators. It has become difficult to tell the difference between information and salesmanship. Conflicts-of-interest abound in this relationship. Two examples make the point.

UnitedHealth. As the debate over health care reform gained momentum in the spring of 2009, UnitedHealth released its proposal to "cut costs". Drafted by its Center for Health Reform and Modernization, it made 15 recommendations that could allegedly save the federal government $540 billion over ten years. These recommendations were mostly speculative, and mostly beyond the direct influence of insurers. The recommendations were cloaked in such non-controversial terms as "providing patients with incentives for going to high-quality, efficient physicians, granting physicians incentives for providing comprehensive and preventive care, and reducing unnecessary care". Projected "savings" included "providing nurse practitioners at nursing homes to manage illness and reduce avoidable hospitalizations ($166 billion), and using evidence-based care management with preventive care to reduce avoidable hospitalizations ($102 billion)." Blue Dog Democrat Mike Ross welcomed this report without skepticism.[33] He became a vocal opponent of the public option and, of course, the single payer option was never on the table.

The Lewin Group's Transformation: From Supplying the Facts to Deep-Sixing the Truth. As a well-known Virginia-based health care consulting group, Lewin has published a number of reports over the last decade showing that, compared to a multi-payer system with any kind of employer and/or individual mandate approach, single payer financing is the only way to provide universal coverage and still save money. The states involved in these studies include California, Connecticut, Georgia, Maryland, Massachusetts and Vermont.[34]

Lewin was bought in 2007 by Ingenix, a subsidiary of UnitedHealth. Lewin prepared a February 2009 report at the request of Blue Cross Blue Shield that could be used to support a single payer system, the policy choice that is anathema to private insurers. It was not released. An online article in *The Washington Post* disclosed Lewin's corporate ties to UnitedHealth and Ingenix.[35] John Sheils, Vice President of the Lewin Group, acknowledged: "Let's just say, sometimes studies come out that don't show exactly what the client wants to see. And in these instances, they have [the] option to bury the study." On the very next day, a followup article in *The Washington Post* by the same reporter on the same subject omitted any reference to Blue Cross Blue Shield, and included this further comment by Sheils: Lewin has gone through a "terribly difficult adjustment" since its purchase by UnitedHealth because corporate ownership "does create the appearance of a conflict-of-interest." In oral testimony before Congressional committees on health reform options, Lewin was silent on the advantages of single payer documented by its earlier studies, and did not bring up its corporate ties until asked.[36]

Involvement with Health Policy Publications

Health Affairs is widely recognized as the leading health policy journal. Established in 1981 and published by Project Hope, it serves as a "multidisciplinary, peer-reviewed journal dedicated to the serious exploration of domestic and international health policy and system change." Its September/October 2009 issue *Bending the Cost Curve* was a special thematic issue focused particularly on the problem of health care inflation and how to address cost containment in the current cycle of health care reform. In an opening introduction, Susan Dentzer, Editor-in-Chief of *Health Affairs*, acknowledged that Aetna, one of the major U.S. insurers, together with the Aetna Foundation, provided lead financial support that *"made this issue possible."*[37] Over the subsequent 200-plus pages, shouldn't we expect to find substantive coverage of a single payer financing option, Medicare-for-All, which is projected to save some $400 billion a year while providing universal coverage of one-tier comprehensive care for all Americans? After looking through the issue, here is all I could find on single payer:

- Out of more than 25 articles, none deal directly with single payer
- The closest any of the articles gets to discussion was in an article by Vladeck and Rice (opening quote of this chapter on market failure) with a short paragraph stating that single payer financing, as a pure monopsony, perhaps works best in controlling health care spending. But the authors quickly went on to say: "Because enacting a single payer system in the United States seems unlikely for the foreseeable future," it's worth considering other cost containment methods, such as better regulating multiple payers.[38]
- Another article highlighting prices as a major cause of health care inflation recognized: "Other nations achieve lower prices by paying for health services through either a single payer or coordinated multi-payers that set or negotiate fees with all providers." The authors answered their own question why we don't do so in this country:

> "National health spending amounts to income for medical care providers, insurers, pharmaceutical companies, medical device manufacturers, and a host of other health care-related industries that profit from the status quo. Efforts to control health care spending consequently threaten the medical care industry's income and trigger fierce resistance."[39]

Behind-the-Scenes Influence of the Foundations: Non-Profits Preserving the Ideological Foundation of For-Profits

The deep pockets of well-established foundations have played a large role over many years in perpetuating our multi-payer for-profit market-based system. It is well known that big conservative foundations such as Koch Family Foundations, the John M. Olin Foundation and the Scaife Family Foundations channel enormous sums of money into right-wing political organizations, multi-million dollar national think tanks, conservative journals, television networks and radio programs.[40] These foundations provide much of the support for such right-wing think tanks as the American Enterprise Institute, the Cato Institute and the National Center for Policy Analysis.

In her excellent book *Invisible Hands: The Making of the Conservative Movement from the New Deal to Reagan*, Kim Phillips-Fein of New York University's Gallatin School traces the evolution of the conservative free-market movement from its roots in the 1930s. As one example of the change from foundation to institute, the American Enterprise Association (AEA) was founded in 1943 by Lewis H. Brown, an entrepreneurial businessman who had struggled to protect the image of business during the New Deal. Funded by such major corporations as General Motors and Ford, the AEA proceeded to carry out "research" that was called into question in 1950 by a congressional committee that found the AEA "hiding behind a self-serving façade of objectivity."[41] In 1962, the AEA changed its name to the American Enterprise Institute for Public Policy Research in order to avoid being confused as a trade association lobbying on behalf of business.[42]

The right-wing think tanks employ full-time "scholars" to publish materials that oppose national health insurance and advocate for privatization, deregulation, health savings accounts, increased cost-sharing and other market-based policies. Together, they serve as a right-wing "echo chamber" carrying out PR functions and masquerading as research organizations.[43]

But what about the so-called more liberal foundations? How do they deal with the single payer option? Unfortunately, while they may posture as working in the public interest, they also are beholden to corporate money and shy away from supporting single payer. These three examples tell the story of how they distance themselves from single payer and drive the health care debate to the center-right:[44]

- *The Public Welfare Foundation.* This foundation gave out grants worth $7 million in 2009-2010, including a $250,000 grant to the Tennessee Health Care Campaign. Its Board of Directors includes a corporate lawyer who represents pharmaceutical, biotechnology, and medical device companies as well as others with close ties to health care interests. When asked about any grants to single payer projects, the foundation's senior program officer for health reform said: "You're barking up the wrong tree here."

- *The Robert Wood Johnson Foundation (RWJ).* With its stated mission (on its Web site) to "improve the health and health care of all Americans," RWJ has funded many grants to encourage incremental tweaks of the present market-based system, but has stringently avoided more fundamental reform. Although RWJ has received many requests for funding of single payer projects, it has never done so.[45] When it does fund some state-based project, it stipulates that it cannot be for single payer. One example is a three-year grant of $750,000 to *Take Action MN*, a Health Care for America NOW! (HCAN) arm in Minnesota that supported the Obama multi-payer plan while discrediting the single payer option as lacking in enough popular support.[46] The Johnson & Johnson trustees include some large GOP donors, some of its executives and others involved with corporate health care. RWJ has also recently aligned itself with a right-wing industry-funded state legislator's group that is crafting legislation at the state level prohibiting both insurance mandates and single payer health care.

- *The Atlantic Philanthropies.* This group of charities with assets of more than $2 billion recently gave a $25 million grant to HCAN, a coalition of many advocacy and labor groups supporting the Administration's multi-payer health care proposal.[47]

These tales may give a sense of hopelessness about what we are up against. But it is important to get as clear a picture as we can of the challenges before us. In later chapters we will find reasons to be optimistic that single payer is not just possible, but essential if we are ever to fix our health care system.

CORPORATE POWER VS. THE PUBLIC TRUST

Wendell Potter, for many years a communications officer for Cigna, one of the country's largest insurers, was forced by his conscience in 2008 to blow the whistle on the industry's many devious practices. Now a Senior Fellow on Health Care for the Center for Media and Democracy, he reminds us of the industry's successful tactics to kill the Clinton Health Plan (CHP) 15 years ago "by using shills and front groups to spread lies and disinformation to scare Americans away from the very reform that would benefit them most." In a recent talk at the Center for American Progress, he recounted many of these tactics:

- Financing of the Health Leadership Council, which spearheaded a coordinated effort to scare the public and members of Congress away from the CHP.
- Buoyed by their success in derailing the CHP, the industry next formed the Health Benefits Coalition; it was set up and run out of one of Washington's biggest PR firms, and played a leading role in successfully killing a move in Congress to pass a Patients' Bill of Rights.
- In the late 1990s, the industry formed the Coalition for Affordable Quality Healthcare in an attempt to improve the image of managed care.
- When lawyers started to bring class-action suits against the industry on behalf of doctors and patients, the industry responded by funding another group, America's Health Insurers, again created and run out of a Washington, D.C.-based PR firm.

More recently, the industry continued with these tactics by discrediting Michael Moore's 2007 movie *Sicko.* Another front group, Health Care America, was established to demonize the health care systems in other countries portrayed in the movie.[48]

Working mainly through large PR firms, the industry utilized all kinds of approaches, including feeding talking points to conservatives in the media and in Congress, linkages to right-wing think tanks, advertising campaigns, mobilizing grassroots and grasstops campaigns, and providing "information" to members of Congress. Typical messages to the public were the same as those being used today, such as warnings against a "government takeover" of the U.S. health care system.

As the insurance industry has carried out these attacks against any efforts to rein in costs and reform health care, its greed boggles the mind. Potter notes that their medical loss ratios (MLRs: what they "lose" by paying for health care services) went from about 5 percent of premium income in 1990 to at least 20 percent today—now amounting to almost a quarter of a *trillion* dollars a year![49] Some insurers have been so effective at cherry-picking the market that they have "achieved" MLRs as low as 70 percent.[50]

Efforts to consolidate corporate power and squelch dissent continue, and were even accelerated by a ruling of the U.S. Supreme Court in January 2010. In the case *Citizens United v. FEC*, the Court ruled that corporations have a First Amendment right to spend unlimited amounts of money to influence the outcomes of elections. By a 5-4 margin the Roberts court overruled two previous decisions upholding the power of Congress to restrict corporate speech during political campaigns.[51] As Katrina vanden Heuvel editorialized in an October 2009 issue of *The Nation* when this case was pending: "If it does so, it will leave the voting process even more vulnerable to capture by the wealthy and powerful."[52]

We have seen a wild battle for revenue in a new "reformed" health care system among and between corporate stakeholders, sometimes even between members of the same industry group. Thus the insurance industry was attacking physicians' high fees as the major reason for inflating health care costs,[53] blaming patients as the cause of increasing insurance premiums,[54] and starting to feud among themselves (e.g. Blue Cross Blue Shield, which markets mainly to the individual market vs. Aetna, a leading player in the large employer-based group market.)[55] Meanwhile, organized medicine was fighting against a larger role of government in health care even as it lobbied for higher Medicare reimbursement, and some proposed changes in reimbursement were pitting specialists against primary care physicians.[56]

So health care "reform" is all about redistribution of money, and is therefore unlikely to result in health care that is more affordable for patients and their families. The way things are going, the only winners will be corporate stakeholders, once again trumping the public interest, as illustrated by Figure 2.2.

In the next chapters we will examine various ways in which corporate interests manipulate the political discourse in an effort to preserve the status quo, starting with how the issues and policy alternatives are framed.

FIGURE 2.2

No Solutions in Sight

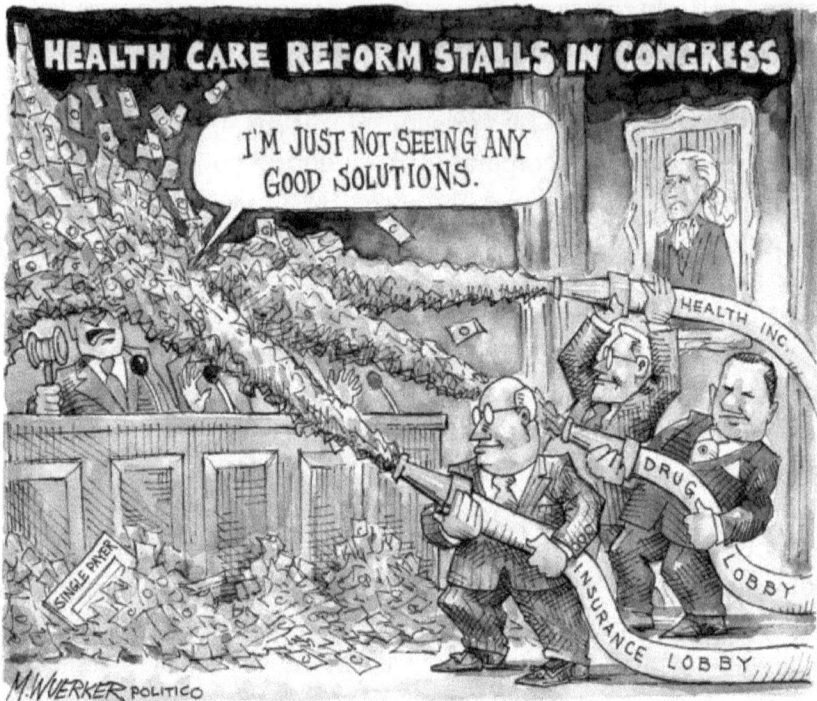

Source: Reprinted with permission of Matt Wuerker of *Politico.*

References

1. Vladeck, B, Rice, T. Market failure and the failure of discourse: Facing up to the power of sellers. *Health Affairs* 28 (5): 1314, 2009.
2. Salant, JD, O'Leary, L. Six lobbyists per lawmaker work on health overhaul. Bloomberg News, as cited in *Truthout*, August 17, 2009.
3. Kroll, A. Lobbyists still run Washington. *The Progressive Populist*, October 15, 2009.
4. Eaton, J, Pell, MB. Lobbyists swarm capitol to influence health reform. Washington, D.C. The Center for Public Integrity, February 23, 2010.
5. Adamy, J, Williamson, E. As Congress goes on break, health lobbying heats up. *Wall Street Journal*, August 5, 2009: A1.
6. Editorial. Puppets in Congress. *New York Times*, November 17, 2009: A28.
7. Ibid # 5.

8. Meropol, NJ, Schulman, KA. Cost of cancer care: Issues and implications. *J Clin Oncology* 25: 180-6, 2007.

9. Bustillo, M, Adamy, J. Trade group challenges Wal-Mart on health care. *Wall Street Journal*, July 13, 2009: A3.

10. Zajak, A. Familiar faces among health industry lobbyists. *Los Angeles Times*, December 21, 2009.

11. The Sunlight Foundation. Visualizing the health care lobbyist complex as featured on NPR's *All Things Considered*/Dollar politics, July 23, 2009. Accessed at http://www.sunlightfoundation.com/projects/2009/healthcare_1...

12. Ibid # 2.

13. Ibid #5.

14. Wedel, J. *Shadow Elite: How the World's New Power Brokers Undermine Democracy, Government, and the Free Market*. New York. Basic Books, 2009.

15. Kirkpatrick, DD. Intended to rein in lobbyists, law sends them underground. *New York Times*, January 18, 2009.

16. Cummings, J. When D.C. rumors move markets. *Politico*, January 19, 2010.

17. Watzman, N. Every dollar is crucial: Washington insiders must play to pay. *Harper's Magazine*, June 2009: 48-9.

18. Ibid # 6.

19. Eggen, D. Industry is generous to influential bloc. *Washington Post* on-line, August 1, 2009.

20. Sirota, D. Thirteen in Congress control health care debate. *Truthout*, August 3, 2009.

21. Ibid # 14.

22. Terhune, C, Epstein, K. Why health insurers are winning. *Business Week*, August 17, 2009: 036.

23. Ibid # 17.

24. Ibid # 2.

25. Ibid # 16.

26. Ibid # 3.

27. Ibid # 15.

28. Connor, K. Chief health aide to Baucus is former Wellpoint executive. *Eyes on the Ties* Blog, September 1, 2009.

29. Connor, K. Wellpoint lobbyist and ex-Enzi staffer write key parts of Baucus plan. *Eyes on the Ties* blog, September 11, 2009.

30. Moyers, B, Winship, M. In Washington, the revolving door is hazardous to your health. *Truthout*, October 11, 2009.

31. Jones, S. Dick Gephardt's spectacular sellout. *The Nation* 289 (12): 24, October 15, 2009.

32. Ibid # 10.

33. Kaiser Daily Health Policy Report, May 28, 2009.

34. Geyman, JP. *The Corrosion of Medicine: Can the Profession Reclaim its Moral Legacy?* Monroe, ME. Common Courage Press. 2008, p 192.

35. Hilzenrath, DS. Research firm cited by GOP is owned by health insurer. *The Washington Post*, July 22, 2009.

36. Hilzenrath, DS. Insurer-owned consulting firm often cited in health debate. *The Washington Post*, July 23, 2009.
37. Dentzer, S. Rolling the rock up the mountain. *Health Affairs* 28 (5): 1250-2, 2009.
38. Ibid # 1.
39. Oberlander, J, White, J. Public attitudes toward health care spending aren't the problem; prices are. *Health Affairs* 28 (5): 1289-91, 2009.
40. People for the American Way. *Buying a Movement: Right-Wing Foundations and American Politics*, 1996. Available at httpa;//www.pfaw.org/media-center/publications/buying-movement
41. Rosenfeld, S. From lobbyists to scholars, 21-30;Smith, JA. *The Idea Brokers: Think Tanks and the Rise of the New Policy Elite*. New York. Free Press, 1991, 175; Report of the Select Committee on Lobbying Activities, House of Representatives, 81st Congress, 2nd sess., Dec. 1950, 19-20, Box 11, GRA, Columbia.
42. Phillips-Fein, K. *Invisible Hands: The Making of the Conservative Movement from the New Deal to Reagan*. New York. W.W. Norton, pp 58-66, 2009.
43. PNHP staff. Right-wing "think" tanks and health policy. The National Health Program Reader. Leadership Training Institute. Chicago, IL, October 24, 2008, p 363.
44. Gray, C. Funding information for single payer from 3 major health care foundations. Unpublished memorandum. Physicians for a National Health Program, April 16, 2010.
45. Hellander, I. Executive Director of Physicians for a National Health Program. Personal communication, November 2, 2009.
46. Sullivan, K. Personal communication, April 17, 2010.
47. Wilhelm, I. Atlantic philanthropies stakes $25-million on health care lobbying group. *The Atlantic Philanthropies*, August 17, 2009.
48. Potter, W. Corporate P.R. is hazardous to your health. The Progressive Populist 15(18), October 15, 2009.
49. Palast, G. The S-word and Dr. Kevorkian's accountant. *Truthout*, October 15, 2009.
50. Terhune, C. New insurance plan has novel pitch – get sick, buy more. *Wall Street Journal*, September 14, 2007: B1.
51. Cullen, J. Editorial. Money talks politics. *The Progressive Populist*, February 15, 2010, p2.
52. vanden Heuvel, K. When money talks. *The Nation* 289 (10): 3,October 5, 2009.
53. Kolata, G. Survey finds high fees common in medical care. *New York Times* on line, August 12, 2009.
54. Beebe, P. Regence campaign: Consumers must make choices to reduce health care costs. *Salt Lake Tribune*, October 14, 2009.
55. Johnson, A, Adamy, J. Signs of a split emerge in insurance industry. *Wall Street Journal*, October 15, 2009: A6.
56. Adamy, J. Doctors fight penalty for heavy test use. *Wall Street Journal*, October 2, 2009: A5.

CHAPTER 3

Who Framed Health Care Reform?
How the Public Was Misled on Issues
and Policy Alternatives

"The election of 2008 was not about small issues. It was nothing less than a battle for America. Despite the imperfections of the nominating and electoral process, the excesses of the media, and the failure to plumb below the surface of the greatest issues confronting America, the election of 2008 was as significant as the nation has experienced at least since 1980, if not 1932 and the advent of the New Deal. At the end, the election was defined by the greatest economic crisis since the Great Depression, raising even greater challenges for the American people and their political system."

—Dan Balz of the *Washington Post* and Haynes Johnson, Pulitzer Prize
author, *The Battle for America: The Story of an Extraordinary Election*[1]

Obama had won with a margin of almost 10 million votes—53 percent of the popular vote—the highest of any Democrat since Lyndon B. Johnson. The electoral college results ended up with 375 for Obama and 163 for McCain. These results were comparable with those of Bill Clinton in 1992 and 1996, all the more remarkable for a northerner and the first African-American president. In a rejection of eight years' of Republican leadership, the Democrats swept both houses of Congress as well as the White House. It appeared to many in this country and around the world that a major transformational change had taken place, a tectonic shift in American politics. Shortly after the election results were announced, President Obama addressed some 70,000 supporters in an outdoor rally in Chicago's Grant Park with these words:

"Change has come. This is our moment. This is our time… to reclaim the American Dream and reaffirm that fundamental truth – that out of many, we are one; that while we breathe, we hope, and where we are met with cynicism, and doubt, and those who tell us that we can't, we will respond with that timeless creed that sums up the spirit of a people: yes, we can."[2]

America seemed destined to set out in new directions, both abroad and at home. Describing the Chicago acceptance speech, Judy Woodruff, PBS News-Hour Senior Correspondent said: "There's a reverence that's taken effect among the thousands of people here… it's a moment of awe. People here know they are witnessing history." News-Hour analyst Mark Shields added: "Americans will look at their country differently tomorrow." And David Brooks, *New York Times* columnist, noted: "In 50 years when people write textbooks this will be the first page of a chapter. A chapter ended and a chapter of some sort is beginning."[3]

So what happened after this supposedly momentous change in America, and what will it mean for health care reform? The last two chapters showed how corporate power and money mobilized rapidly and subverted much of a reform agenda. But there were still other factors at work, including how the issues and policy alternatives were framed in the first place by both political parties.

How health care issues are framed not only determines the possibilities and outcomes of reform efforts, but also defines the character and values of the society. As T. R. Reid, correspondent for the *Washington Post* and author of the book *The Healing of America: A Global Quest for Better, Cheaper and Fairer Health Care*, has noted:

"The design of any country's health care system involves political, medical and economic decisions. But the primary issue for any health care system is, as President Obama made clear last week, a moral question: should a rich society provide health care to everyone who needs it? If a nation answers yes to that moral question, it will build a health care system like the ones in Britain, Germany, Canada, France and Japan, where everyone is covered. If a nation doesn't decide to provide universal coverage, then you're likely to end up with a system where some people get the finest medical care on earth in the finest hospitals, and tens of thousands of others are left to die for lack of care. Without the moral commitment, in other words, you end up with a system like America's."[4]

Framing is not just an abstract academic exercise, but has everything to do with whether reform initiatives can be successful or not. If a necessary policy alternative does not fall within the frames of the policy debate, it will be excluded from consideration and action. Instead, misguided framing will beget misguided approaches to "reform", which many will not recognize as illusory and ineffective. Then obviously, when the best solutions are off the table, the problems requiring reform only get worse.

In order to better understand how health care reform has been framed during and after the 2008 elections, and how we can re-frame the health care debate in the public interest, this chapter undertakes three goals: (1) to compare framing of health care issues by Democrats and Republicans; (2) to show how both of these frames have missed widely accepted target policy objectives; and (3) to suggest how an evidence-based approach informed by health policy science can re-frame the debate over policy alternatives.

HOW HAS HEALTH CARE REFORM BEEN FRAMED?

The Democrats: Killing Hope for Real Reform

With control of the Executive Branch and both chambers of Congress that were for a time immune to Republican filibuster, the Democrats held the power to frame the issues and push health care reform in the public interest. Despite this advantage, they failed on framing right out of the starting gate.

Instead of taking a forceful approach to the well-known problems of the health care system, including the widely recognized surging costs of health care, decreasing access and obsolescence of a failing private insurance industry,[5] the Democratic starting position on reform was overly moderate, discarding the only progressive approach to real reform—replacement of a failing, inefficient and exploitive private health insurance industry by a publicly-financed national health insurance program.

Disguised as a middle-of-the-road approach, the Democrats took a pro-industry position at the expense of Americans. These are the main tenets that Democrats advanced to reform health care:

- Keep your insurance if you like it.
- Build on our system's many strengths, we don't need to rebuild it entirely.
- Increase choice by offering a public option to private insurance, with the intent on "keeping insurers honest."

In effect, then, Democrats sought an approach that favored the interests of existing private industry. Hoping for bipartisan support, they made a political calculation that a single payer system was not politically feasible, thereby narrowing the debate to one question: how should we work with private interests to address health care problems? In effect, this was a Surrender-in-Advance strategy that killed their hopes of real reform.

This approach was no accident. It had been carefully worked out over several years by various groups. The Herndon Alliance, for example, is a coalition formed in 2005 including liberal health care groups, labor unions and patient-advocacy groups, convened to develop a new language to promote universal health care. They brought on Celinda Lake, self-described as one of the Democratic party's "leading political strategists", to help frame their message. She went through a three-stage "research" process (without transparency of her methods) that claimed to find that single payer lacked meaningful public support. One example of her deceptive methods: in the polling stage, she offered respondents two choices—asking them whether they favored "guaranteed affordable choice" or single payer. But she declined to clarify that the "guaranteed affordable choice" would have in fact limited the choice of physicians and hospitals vs. complete freedom of choice of both under single payer. Here are some of her bogus "findings":

- "Americans think Medicare is "frighteningly flawed" and, consequently, Americans oppose a national health insurance program based on Medicare or that resembles Medicare;
- Americans who have private health insurance not only like it, but like it so much they will resist a Medicare-for-all solution to the health care crisis because it does not leave them the option of continuing to receive coverage from a health insurance company;

- Americans don't want to pay for health insurance for "the undeserving," a category which includes even the parents of average Americans;
- Americans don't like the phrase "universal coverage" or "universal health insurance," and prefer "quality, affordable health care;"
- Similarly, activists should never say "Medicare for all" and instead say "choice of public and private plans," which is, of course, equivalent to saying no one should support a Medicare-for-all (or single payer bill) and should instead only support legislation that allows the health insurance industry to continue to take in tax dollars and premium payments."[6,7]

These "results" contradicted dozens of legitimate national studies and surveys over many years showing that 65 to 85 percent of Americans support universal health insurance, and that 60 to 70 percent support a Medicare-for-all program.[8]

Because the Democratic party leadership opposed single payer, they leapt on any pseudo evidence they could find to denigrate or marginalize single payer. Another coalition, Health Care for America NOW! (HCAN), a labor-consumer coalition of some 30 groups, including the AFL-CIO, the Service Employees International Union (SEIU), USAction, MoveOn.org and La Raza, actually attacked the single payer approach based on Celinda Lake's focus groups and dubious polling. The SEIU also participated in a broad "affordable choice" alliance favoring only modest change of our existing multi-payer financing system. These groups ranged from the American Medical Association and American Hospital Association to America's Health Insurance Plans, corporations such as Wal-Mart and Intel, the U.S. Chamber of Commerce, and the conservative Business Roundtable.[9]

President Obama accepted this centrist approach, a complete flip-flop from his position on single payer as a candidate several years earlier. Speaking to the Illinois AFL-CIO, he had this to say about single payer in 2003:

"I happen to be a proponent of a single payer universal health care program... (applause)... I see no reason why the United States of America, the wealthiest country in the history of the world, spending 14 percent of its Gross National Product on health care, cannot provide basic health insurance to everybody. And that's what Jim is talking about when he says everybody in, nobody out. A single payer health care plan, a universal health care plan. And that's what I'd like to see. But as all of you know, we may not get there immediately. Because first we have to take back the White House, we have to take back the Senate, and we have to take back the House."[10]

Whereas Obama the candidate later acknowledged that he would propose single payer "if I were starting from scratch", as president he bought into the view that it was politically infeasible. That led Republicans to believe they could dilute or even kill health care reform altogether. And as a furious debate erupted over a public option (a watered-down poor substitute for single payer potentially open to only a few million Americans), he even refused to draw a line in the sand over that, describing it as "just a sliver" of his reform plan.[11] Meanwhile, he deferred the task of working through the details of reform to Congress.

The Republicans: Is There a Word Doctor in the House?

Frank Luntz, political consultant and pollster, gives us a good example of how the Republican message machine works. His current company, The Word Doctors, "specializes in message creation and image management for commercial and political clients", is a good example of how the Republican message machine works. When interviewed by PBS Frontline, Luntz described his specialty as "testing language and finding words that will help his clients sell their product or turn public opinion on an issue or a candidate." He has authored two recent books: *Words That Work: It's Not What You Say, It's What People Hear* (2007) and *What Americans Really Want...Really* (2009).[12]

As the health care debate intensified in the spring of 2009, Luntz delivered a confidential (soon to become public) 26-page report to Capitol Hill Republicans warning that Americans want health care reform, and that legislators must avoid an appearance of being against reform. As he said: "You simply MUST be vocally and passionately on the side of REFORM. The status quo is no longer acceptable. If the dynamic becomes 'President Obama is on the side of reform and Republicans are against it,' then the battle is lost and every word in this document is useless. Republicans must be for the right kind of reform that protects the quality of health care for all Americans." He further recommended 10 rules for stopping the "Washington Takeover" of health care (Table 3.1).[13]

One month after Luntz circulated his recommendations to

TABLE 3.1

Luntz's 10 Rules for Stopping the "Washington Takeover" of Healthcare

1. Humanize your approach.
2. Acknowledge the "crisis" or suffer the consequences.
3. "Time" is the government health care killer.
4. The arguments against the Democrats' healthcare plan must center around "politicians", "bureaucrats", and "Washington"... not the free market, tax incentives, or competition.
5. The health care denial horror stories from Canada & Co. do resonate, but you have to humanize them.
6. Health care quality = "getting the treatment you need, when you need it."
7. "One-size-does-NOT-fit-all." WASTE, FRAUD, and ABUSE are your best targets for how to bring down costs.
8. Americans will expect the government to look out for those who truly can't afford health care.
9. It's not enough to just say what you're against.
10. You have to tell them what you're for.

Source: Luntz, F. The Language of Healthcare 2009. As cited in Allen, M. Luntz to GOP: Health care is popular. *Politico*, May 5, 2009.

Congressional Republicans, the Sunlight Foundation reported the following increases in usage of these words in the Congressional Record:

- "rationing" – 18 to 90 uses
- "doctor-patient" – 6 to 20 uses
- "takeover" – 13 to 106 uses
- "bureaucrats" – 53 to 78 uses[14]

These words, as recommended by Luntz's fourth rule, were intended to spread fear of a larger role of the government in health care policy. Shortly thereafter the GOP message man sent a memo to fellow Republican strategists recommending new language for them to use in the health care debate. Here are some excerpts: "It's time to look at health care reform in a new way. The President sees the problem. So do we. He talks of making health care more affordable. So do we. But we have a completely different vision of how to fix it."

Without suggesting any specific proposals, the memo continues:

"We support *patient-centered reforms.*"
"We want common-sense *simple fixes* that will yield real results."
"The patient-centered health care movement supports *an open health-care system* where patients and doctors make health care decisions."
"We want a *bottom-up, patient-centered system* where control remains with your doctor and you."
"We want to *get politics out of health care* not put more politics in. We want *common sense fixes not politically driven experiments.*"
"*The Obama Experiment* with our health could change everything we like about our health care – and our economy. ... President Obama is experimenting with America, *too much, too soon, and too fast.* ... Slow down, Mr. President. We can't afford to get health care wrong."[15]

Note that all of these statements are rhetorical only, lacking in any substantive ideas for health care reform.

Then, during the Congressional summer recess as the GOP was fomenting so many angry discussions against the "Obama experiment" in town halls across the country, Republican National Committee Chairman Michael Steele released a "Seniors Health Care Bill of Rights" opposing any efforts by the government to trim Medicare spending or limit end-of-life care for Medicare beneficiaries. The manifesto vowed to fight any Democratic move to "ration care or to insert the government between seniors and their doctors."[16] This is especially cynical in view of the long-standing effort by Republicans to shrink Medicare as an entitlement program, and its apparent tacit approval to continue subsidized overpayments to private Medicare plans that have not been found by independent non-partisan studies to add to the value of seniors' care. The irony of the Republicans' new gambit to defend seniors against the evils of "government-run health care" is captured in Figure 3.1.[17]

Many critics across the political spectrum were dubious, correctly so, that the health care bills being touted by many Democrats and the Obama Administration would actually be effective in containing health care costs. Sensing Obama's vulnerability on this critical point, conservative political analyst William Kristol had this recommendation:

> "With ObamaCare on the ropes, there will be a temptation for opponents to let up on their criticism, and try to appear constructive, or at least responsible. There will be a tendency to want to let the Democrats' plans sink of their own weight, to emphasize that the critics have been pushing sound reform ideas all along and suggest it's not too late for a bipartisan compromise over the next couple of weeks or months. My advice, for what it's worth: Resist the temptation. This is no time to pull punches. Go for the kill."[18]

Kristol and his fellow conservatives were right, but for the wrong reasons, as will be discussed further in a later chapter—right that the

FIGURE 3.1

A Sense of Irony?

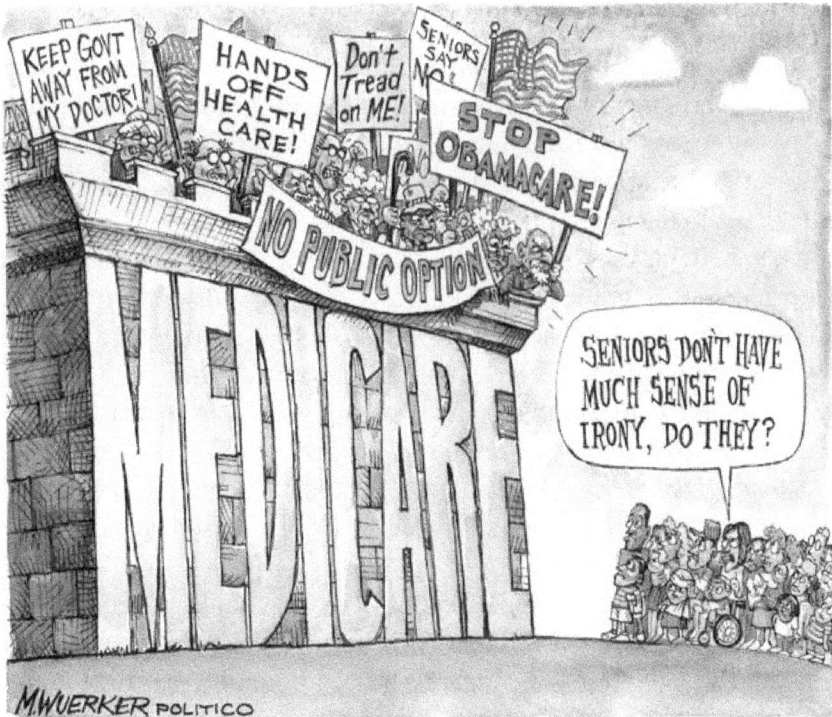

Source: Reprinted with permission of Matt Wuerker of *Politico.*

bills wouldn't sufficiently rein in costs, but wrong because they involved too much government intervention.

HOW BOTH FRAMES WERE OFF TARGET

The frames advanced by the right and by the left both failed to inform useful policy alternatives to address our growing system problems of cost, access and quality of health care. They both shared in common a reason for this failure—they were not focused on our major system problems and they were not informed by the track record of previous incremental reform attempts. Both seemed unaware of health policy science. And they also differed in this way: Republican framing was largely distorted or untrue, based on ideology and scare words, while Democratic framing was dominated by political considerations. Democrats attempted to sell their version of reform on the basis that "you can keep your insurance"—a maneuver that would keep single payer off the table—even when Obama and many others knew that single payer was the best reform option.

Framing by the right was aimed to defend the status quo, asserting that free markets can fix our problems and that free enterprise and individual responsibility are core American values which serve us better than a larger role of government. While offering no substantive policy alternatives, Republicans attempted to hijack the values discussion with assertions that were often totally false. For example, conservatives latched on to a falsehood that ObamaCare would set up "death panels" as part of its Medicare cutbacks.[19] That was in reference to a provision (Section 1233) in H.R. 3200, the House bill that called for Medicare coverage of *voluntary* counseling discussions with one's physician about end-of-life planning, such as living wills—hardly death panels. Conservatives also demagogued projected cutbacks of Medicare Advantage overpayments, private Medicare plans that are subsidized by overpayments of 13 percent or more compared to traditional Medicare without demonstrating increased value of their coverage.[20]

As previously discussed, Republican approaches to health care, although claimed by the right to be congruent with American values, are quite the contrary. Compared to traditional American values of efficiency, choice, fiscal responsibility, equity and integrity, for example, conservative pro-market health care policies go in exactly the opposite direction as they value private profits over public service, often at the expense of the public.[21] Lost in the right's arguments are the facts—for example, patients in private Medicare plans have *less* choice of physicians and hospitals than those covered by traditional Medicare; and Medicare as a government-run single payer system is bound legally to provide a comprehensive set of benefits for all beneficiaries, hardly the case with private insurers who regularly deny claims, rescind coverage, or even leave their market if their revenues are not sufficient.

The modus operandi employed by Luntz in the health care debate seems to be the standard issue of opposition tactics. He later used the same tactics against financial regulation of Wall Street, as illustrated by Paul Krugman's commentary some months later. Luntz had distributed a memo in January 2010 to the Republican leadership on how best to combat financial reform. His main recommendation was: "The single best way to kill any legislation is to link it to the Big Bank Bailout". Dutifully, Mitch McConnell (R-KY), as Senate Minority Leader, later pretended to stand up for taxpayers while in fact doing exactly the opposite. He and other GOP leaders had been meeting for some time with Wall Street executives and lobbyists in an effort to coordinate their political strategy as they worked toward ways to deprive regulators in the future of tools needed to seize failing financial firms.[22] The analogy to GOP tactics on health care is stark: by posturing as defenders of seniors against government cutbacks, the GOP was saying in both instances the exact opposite of what they were trying to achieve.

Terrified as conservative politicians are about a single payer financing system of national health insurance, they go out of their way to denigrate the Canadian single payer system as antithetical to American values. In their attacks on public financing, conservatives argue that choice will be limited by public financing (absolutely untrue, as the Medicare example above shows), that public financing is un-American (are Medicare and the Veterans Administration un-American?), and that public financing inherently involves greater bureaucracy than private financing (our private health insurance industry has a workforce 10 to 25 times larger than that of the Canadian single payer system.)[23]

A fascinating rebuttal to conservative fears about the Canadian system was given by Dr. Sherif Emil, pediatric surgeon for many years at the University of California Irvine. After moving to Canada to practice in 2008, he was invited back by the graduating medical students to give the 2010 Commencement Address at that medical school. Here is what he said at the time:

"It was interesting to me, as an American physician practicing in Canada, to see the recent negative depictions of the Canadian system in TV ads and lay media, depictions that bore absolutely no resemblance to the actual environment in which I practice daily. My reality is very different. I can see any patient and any patient can see me—total freedom of practice. My patients' parents have peace of mind regarding their children's health. If they change jobs or lose their job altogether in a bad economy, their children will still get the same care and see the same physicians. Micromanagement of daily practice has become a thing of the past for me. There are no contracts, authorizations, denials, appeals, reviews, forms to complete, IPAs, HMOs, or PPOs. Our Division's billing overhead is 1%. My relationship with the hospital administration is defined by professional, not financial, standards. I have no allegiance to any corporate or government entity, nor does one ever get in between me and the patient. This environment, which some denigrate as the ever so scary system of "socialized medicine" allows for more patient autonomy and choice than was available to most of my patients in California."[24]

Conservative rhetoric beats a steady drumbeat that the U.S. is uniquely different from other advanced countries that have established one or another form of publicly-financed health insurance, and that such a system could never happen in this country. But as T. R. Reid points out, the myth of "American exceptionalism"—that we have nothing to learn from the experience of other countries because we are so unique—is losing sway in this country as more Americans are coming to realize that other countries are getting more and better health care for less money than we do.[25] The desperate strategies of the right have even come under intense criticism. For example, Oregon Democrat Jeff Merkley made this impassioned speech on the floor of the Senate admonishing the Republican Minority Leader Mitch McConnell for taking Luntz's health care talking points and running with them:

"My friends, it is irresponsible in the face of 50 million Americans without health care, with working Americans in every one of our states going bankrupt as they struggle with health care expenses. It's irresponsible to utilize a road map of rhetoric that comes from polling about how to scare people. That's irresponsible."[26]

Framing on the left, while mostly non-distortional, has been timid in not rising up against the basic problem of increasing costs and decreasing access to health care—the profiteering by corporate stakeholders in the medical-industrial complex. Many on the left seem unable or unwilling to acknowledge that market failure is at the root of our cost and access problems, as well as the variable quality of care that goes with perverse incentives toward provision of more services, whether or not medically indicated or appropriate. Democrats have been unwilling to join the fight. They fail to answer conservative value-based assertions, even though that argument can be well made on the evidence. For example, single payer public financing of health care fits closely with all of our closely-held traditional American values, including efficiency, choice, fiscal responsibility, opportunity, equity, integrity, and accountability.

Some voices and a few groups, however, rang true and clear. In his new book, *Obama's Challenge*, Robert Kuttner, founder and co-editor of *The American Prospect* and co-founder of the Economic Policy Institute, argues that any reform short of single payer will only worsen our problems:

"The assumption that a single, comprehensive system is politically out of the question puts America on a path that would combine nominal universal coverage with deterioration in what is actually covered, plus acceleration of cost-shifting to individuals."[27]

Kuttner is shining a light toward the change we voted for, a subject we will return to in Part III of this book.

AN HONEST FRAMEWORK
AS A PREREQUISITE TO THE WAY FORWARD

Framing of health care reform must draw from moral, social and economic perspectives. Health care should not be just another commodity for sale as it has become in our market-based system. Everyone should have a right to necessary health care, as captured by the notions "Everybody In, Nobody Out" and "Medicare for All". From a social perspective, we are a stronger and healthier society if we are all in the same boat (as we are concerning risk of disease and injury). And from an economic perspective, we (like all other nations) do not have unlimited resources, and have to decide how to best allocate what resources we have. So far we allocate based on ability to pay, a cruel kind of rationing imposed on lower-income people, instead of allocating based on medical need.

Health care and health insurance are basic human needs, and should not be framed on an ideological or partisan basis. Concerning whether we should finance health care through a multi-payer, mostly for-profit and investor-owned system or a single payer not-for-profit public system, it makes sense to apply traditional American values to that policy decision. If we do so, single payer wins hands down in assuring universal access to necessary health care for our entire population, being the most efficient and fair, and offering the most choice, opportunity and reliability of coverage. The entire debate over health care reform can be captured by the following simple formulation:

> "Restore the promise of opportunity and security by promoting better health of our people, communities and country through enlightened health policies of fiscal prudence and fairness to all."[28]

In their 2007 Rockridge Institute Report on *The Logic of the Health Care Debate*, George Lakoff and his colleagues called for government to assert its moral responsibility to empower and protect its citizens. They also identified these progressive requirements for a just health care system:

- "Everyone should have access to comprehensive, quality health care.
- No one should be denied care for the sake of private profit.
- You can choose your own doctor.
- Promotion of health and well-being, focusing on preventive care.
- Costs should be progressive, that is, readily affordable to everyone, with higher costs borne by those better able to pay.

- Access should be extremely easy, with no specific roadblocks.
- Administration should be simple and cheap.
- Interactions should be minimally bureaucratic and maximally human.
- Payments should be adequate for doctors, nurses, and other health care workers.
- When people are harmed by either the unsafe practices or negligence of health care providers, the redress should be left to the courts—with no arbitrary caps on compensatory payments."[29]

In an important article in the *New England Journal of Medicine,* Dr. Akkab Brett, from his base at the University of South Carolina School of Medicine, describes how much of the conservative rhetoric about health care reform hides behind a smoke screen of "American values" with the unfounded claim that single payer financing is antithetical to our traditional values. He suggests this approach to counter the claims by conservatives that American individualism and uniqueness do not solve our health care problems:

> "In an increasingly diverse country that has a widening gap between rich and poor, a more promising approach is to start with the questions that matter to everyone: Will the system care for us when we're sick and help prevent illness when we're well? Will we have access to medical care throughout our lives without risking financial ruin? Will we be able to navigate the system easily, without jumping through unnecessary hoops or encountering excessive red tape? Will health care spending be managed wisely?"[30]

These value-based questions give us a useful way to envision our goals and define our criteria as to how best to reform our system. Common sense tells us to consider the history of previous reform attempts, and then to focus our policy alternatives on the major problems of the system. Table 3.2 (next page) shows how we can do this with regard to a financing system. As we can see, single payer NHI can directly address problems of cost, affordability, access and quality by providing a simplified more accountable financing system upon which to build more effective approaches to other system problems, such as moving toward payment reform, a more evidence-based approach

TABLE 3.2

A Problem-Oriented Approach to System Reform

PROBLEM	ACTION
1. Uncontrolled inflation of health care costs and prices	Advocate for single-payer National Health Insurance (NHI), Medicare for All, a publicly financed program of comprehensive health insurance coupled with a private delivery system; lower overhead and improved efficiency by risk pooling across our entire population. NHI would consolidate health care programs, simplify administration, and provide the structure for more accountability to the system.
2. Growing crisis in unaffordability of health care now extending to middle class	
3. Decreasing access to care	
4. Rising rates of uninsured and underinsured	
5. Gaps in coverage for essential services	
6. 29-month waiting period for coverage of disabled on Medicare	
7. Lack of mental health parity	
8. Discontinuity and turnover of insurance coverage	
9. Variable, often poor quality of care	
10. High rates of inappropriate and unnecessary care	
11. Increasing health disparities	
12. Administrative complexity, profiteering and waste of 1,300 private insurers	
13. Decreased choice of hospital and physician in managed care programs	
14. Erosion of safety net programs	
15. Lax federal regulation of drug, medical device, and dietary supplement industries	Advocate for expanded authority and resources for FDA and support its independence from political interference.
16. Inadequate national system for assessment of new medical technologies	Support creation of new federal agency for this purpose, possibly along the lines of the National Transportation Safety Board.
17. Declining primary care base	Support narrowing of reimbursement gap between procedural and cognitive health care services, together with other policies to expand training programs and strengthen the delivery model for primary care physicians.

Source: Reprinted with permission from Geyman, JP, *The Corrosion of Medicine: Can the Profession Reclaim Its Moral Legacy?* Monroe, ME. Common Courage Press, 2008, p 216.

to decisions about adoption of new technologies, and rebuilding our primary care base.

Beyond flawed framing of the issues, there are other important reasons why health care reform went off track. In the next chapter we will look at how competing interests take the distorted frames we have seen here to guide the political debate and outcomes to further their agendas.

References

1. Balz, D, Johnson, H. *The Battle for America 2008*: *The Story of an Extraordinary Election*. New York. Penguin Group, 2009, p 386.
2. Ibid #1.
3. Ibid #1.
4. Reid, T.R. No country for sick men. *Newsweek*, September 21, 2009: 43.
5. Geyman, JP. *Do Not Resuscitate: Why the Health Insurance Industry Is Dying and How We Must Replace It*. Monroe, ME. Common Courage Press, 2008.
6. Sullivan, K. An analysis of Celinda Lake's slide show, :"How to talk to voters about health care." November 29, 2008. Available at http://www.pnhp.org. news.2008/december/americans support si.php
7. All Unions Committee for Single Payer Health Care—H.R. 676. Why does Celinda Lake oppose single payer? Available at http://www.pnhp.org/news/2008/December/why_does_celinda_l...
8. Ibid # 6.
9. Bybee, R. Skewed debate: Strange bedfellows oppose single payer healthcare reform. *In These Times*, 33 (6): 18-9, June 2009.
10. Obama, B. Speech to the Illinois AFL-CIO, June 30, 2003.
11. Nichols, J. If Obama discards the public option, what's left of reform? The Beat. *The Nation*, August 16, 2009.
12. Wikopedia listing for Frank Luntz, accessed September 13, 2009.
13. Luntz, FI, The Language of Healthcare 2009. As cited in Allen, M. Luntz to GOP: Health care is popular. *Politico*, May 5, 2009
14. Tracking the influence of Frank Luntz's obstructionist health care memo. *Think Progress*, July 27, 2009.
15. Castellanos, A. GOP health care talking points. July 7, 2009. As cited by the *Washington Post*, July 20, 2009.
16. King, N. GOP tees up Medicare manifesto. *Wall Street Journal*, August 25, 2009: A4.
17. Wuerker, M. Medicare cartoon. *The Progressive Populist*, October 15, 2009.
18. Kristol, W. Kill it and start over. The Blog. *The Weekly Standard*. July 20, 2009.
19. EIN News. 'Death panel' inventor Betsy McCaughey has close ties to Philip Morris, September 21, 2009.

20. Kaiser Daily Health Policy Report, January 15, 2009.
21. Ibid # 5, p 187.
22. Krugman, P. The fire next time. *New York Times*, April 15, 2010.
23. Woolhandler, S, Campbell, T, Himmelstein, DU. Costs of health care administration in the United States and Canada. *N Engl J Med* 349: 768, 2003.
24. Emil, S. An American in Canada. Commencement Address, University of California Irvine School of Medicine, Irvine, CA, June 5, 2010.
25. Reid, TR. Myths about health care around the world. *Washington Post*, August 23, 2009.
26. Merkeley, J. Stand Up Guy. The Senator takes on talking points. *The Washington Spectator* 35 (17), 1, September 15, 2009.
27. Kuttner, R, as quoted in Bybee, R. Skewed debate. Strange bedfellows oppose single payer healthcare reform. *In These Times* 33 (6): 19, June 2009.
28. Ibid # 5, p 186.
29. Lakeoff, G, Haas, E, Smith, GW, & Parkinson, S. *The Logic of the Health Care Debate.* Berkeley, CA: A Rockridge Institute Report, October 15, 2007.
30. Brett, A. "American values"—A smoke screen in the debate on health care reform. *N Engl J Med* 361 (5): 441, 2009.

CHAPTER 4

The Three D's—
Distortion, Disinformation and Deception:
Their Use by the Left and Right
For and Against Reform

What were the tactics of the left and right? How successful were they in influencing public opinion? Why does the gap between their fictions and the facts matter?

As we saw in the last chapter, both sides of the debate over health care reform made major efforts to frame the issues according to their own interests. Throughout all stages of the political battle in Congress and across the country, we saw how these framings played out in the nation's political discourse. The three D's are closely intertwined with and typically cloaked under deceptive front groups with names suggesting the opposite of their real mission.

In this chapter we will: (1) describe highlights of the campaigns waged by the right and the left to support or oppose health care reform bills as they were being shaped in Congress; (2) summarize their impact on public opinion; and (3) consider how the disconnect between actual and fabricated issues matters in the debate over health care.

LIES, DAMN LIES AND HEALTH CARE
From the Left

In general, the campaign on the left for health care reform was defensive, uncoordinated and ineffective in countering the right's opposition to health care reform. On the left, distortions of information were less frequent. But the left also misrepresented the issues in a number of instances, and some of their claims were not well founded.

As we saw in the last chapter, reformers on the left were timid in framing the main issues, a surrender-in-advance tactic intended to draw broad bipartisan political support. Formerly an advisor to President Bill Clinton during the 1990s, Democratic pollster Celinda Lake drew from the conclusions of the Herndon Alliance that Americans want to keep our multi-payer system and would reject single payer (a point refuted by a large body of poll data that has been consistent over decades). In 2008 she proposed the language to be used by the left to promote reform. She recommended that these terms be eliminated from the debate—"universal health coverage", "public plan" and "single payer"—and replaced by these terms—"guaranteed affordable choice" and "competition."[1]

In an excellent detailed analysis of Lake's linguistic proposal, Kip Sullivan, attorney, health policy expert and author of *The Health Care Mess: How We Got Into It and How We'll Get Out of It*, shows how Lake's suggestions, based as they were on false premises and lack of information, led us astray from the real goals of health care reform.[2]

The Obama Administration and most Democrats put politics above health policy in choosing to base its reform agenda on a failing multi-payer financing system. Lacking the political courage to take on the corporate power brokers of the medical industrial complex, they worked very hard to compromise principle and known health policy science for a project labeled "reform" that would win votes but fail to correct system problems. How else can we account for their failure, with rare exceptions, to even consider putting single payer on the negotiating table?

In a classic example of double talk, in his message to the Democratic caucus in the House 24 hours before the big vote on the Senate bill on March 21, President Obama declared that the Senate bill was the biggest advance in health care legislation since Medicare and Medicaid in 1965. He dismissed single payer as "government-run," without noting that Medicare and Medicaid *are* government-run![3]

From the Right
Conservatives and their allies on the right launched a well funded and coordinated campaign aimed at defeating health care reform, handing the new Administration a resounding defeat early in its term, and building support for the election cycles of 2010 and 2012. The party of No was almost entirely united in this effort, with its messages ranging from a libertarian view that government is the enemy, to the

superiority of free markets to fix problems, the need to safeguard our citizens from higher taxes, and the intrusion of government in our private lives.

In 1997, Rick Scott was fired from his post as CEO of Columbia/ HCA, the largest investor-owned hospital chain in the country, after the chain was found guilty of fraud, settled by $1.7 billion, for such tactics as overbilling Medicare, giving kickbacks to physicians referring patients to its hospitals, and understaffing hospitals to cut costs.[4] Now he has a new passion as founder and head of *Conservatives for Patients' Rights (CPR)*. CPR describes itself on its web site as a "non-profit organization dedicated to educating and informing the public about the principles of patients' rights and, in doing so, advancing the debate over health care reform ... Any serious discussion of health care reform that does not include choice, competition, accountability and responsibility—the four 'pillars' of patients' rights—will result in our government truly becoming a 'nanny-state,' making decisions based on what is best for society and government rather than individuals deciding what is best for each of us."[5] In announcing the formation of CPR on the day after President Obama's first address to Congress, Scott also inaugurated a $20 million campaign to pressure members of Congress to base future health reform proposals on free-market principles.[6] This campaign should give us pause when we consider the sincerity of CPR's commitment to patients.

Dick Armey, former Republican House Majority Leader, believes that "individual liberty and the freedom to compete increases consumer choices and provides individuals with the greatest control over what they own and earn."[7] *FreedomWorks* is a Washington, D.C.-based organization founded in 1984 with a mission to "recruit, educate, train and mobilize hundreds of thousands of volunteer activists to fight for lower taxes, less government and more freedom." As the current head of Freedom Works, Armey hired the same PR firm that ran the notorious Swift Boat Veterans assault of presidential candidate John Kerry in 2004, putting out national television ads stating that ObamaCare will give us "government-run health care."[8] Recall that the Obama plan would *not* be government-run, but would still rely on a private system (as does Medicare). Moreover, the VA health care system *is* a government-run system with generally higher quality of care than its private counterparts.[9-11]

Here are some other organizations created by the right to spread its false and misleading messages:

Americans for Prosperity (AFP) and its ***Foundation*** is a national organization, based in Washington, D.C, with state chapters all around the country. Claiming more than 700,000 members on its web site, its "grassroots" membership "advocate for public policies that champion the principles of entrepreneurship and fiscal and regulatory restraint." Its activities include organizing events, writing letters to editors, and petitioning legislators to "uphold freedom and prosperity."[12] It ran a $3 million advertising campaign to denigrate the Canadian single payer system, featuring an inaccurate story of a Canadian woman named Shona Holmes. She claimed that she had been told she would have to wait six months to be treated for a brain tumor, so she re-mortgaged her house and came to the U.S. for treatment. She was found to have a benign cyst of the brain, not needing immediate care, but still was represented as having survived a brain tumor with the inaccurate claim that she would have died if she had relied on care in Canada.[13]

Health Care America. The health insurance industry created and staffed this group to help counter the impact of Michael Moore's movie, *Sicko,* in an attempt to discredit Moore and to denigrate the health care systems shown in the movie, such as France and Canada. In this effort, it hired a conservative PR firm to warn against "government takeover;" in one ad, it ran this message: "In America, you wait in line to see a movie. In government-run health care systems, you wait to see a doctor."[14]

Club for Growth. According to its web site, this is a national network of thousands of Americans to promote economic growth through such means as making the Bush tax cuts permanent, cutting and limiting government spending, repealing the death tax and replacing our tax code, regulatory reform and deregulation.[15] One ad in its $1.2 million advertising campaign showed a distraught man at his dying wife's bedside as a narrator said: "$22,750. In England, government health officials decided that's how much six months of life is worth … Life and death decisions should be made by patients and doctors, not politicians and bureaucrats."[16]

Council for Affordable Health Insurance (CAHI). On its web site, CAHI describes itself as a "research and advocacy association of insurance carriers in the individual, small group, HSA and senior markets." Its members include insurance companies, insurance brokers, small businesses, providers, individuals and actuaries.[17] One of its latest activities was to lobby for an important detail in health reform legislation—the lowest possible MLR to be required of insurers. Some state regulators set that mark at 70 percent; CAHI would like to see MLRs of 55 to 65 percent, meaning that insurers could keep up to 45 percent of premium revenue for administration, marketing, and profits, claiming that they otherwise could not do business in the non-group market.[18]

The standard message of conservatives on the right and their corporate allies is that they are in favor of health care reform, but not if it raises taxes, increases the deficit, or increases government control over health care. At the same time, stakeholders want to hedge their bets and improve their lot if health "reform" were to happen, leading to some coalitions of strange bedfellows. *Americans for Stable Quality Care* is one such example. Its web site states its mission as advocating for reforms that will "make health care more affordable and stable for all." Its particular aim is to eliminate pre-existing conditions as reasons for denial of insurance coverage. Its supporters include the AMA, the Federation of American Hospitals (which represents investor-owned hospitals), PhRMA, and Families USA.[19]

As we saw in Chapter 1, these groups of physicians, hospitals and the drug industry would likely see a bonanza if health "reform" along the lines of bills in Congress became law. They could expect to see their "pledges" more than repaid from future revenues. It therefore comes as no surprise that this group launched a $12 million television ad campaign targeted at states with Blue Dog Democrats or others opposing or on the fence about reform. This 30-second ad showed smiling patients and providers in an effort to support the idea that a reform bill would make health care more accessible and affordable, lower costs, reform health insurance, and cut waste and red tape.[20] We will see in later chapters how far short of reality those assertions are.

In some instances, some of the above organizations got together to collaborate on joint efforts to advance their case against reform as it was being developed in Congress. One example is the collaboration of *FreedomWorks* and *Conservatives for Patients' Rights* in planning and organizing the disruptive town hall meetings during the summer of 2009 to protest against health care reform plans. As Astroturf, or fake grassroots organizations, they carried these meetings to a whole new level of uncivility, including placing protestors with loaded handguns, or even larger weapons, which turned out to be within the law in some states.[21,22] Another example was the collaboration of **FreedomWorks** and **Americans for Prosperity** in organizing anti-tax "tea party" demonstrations with instructions on how to harass and disrupt the proceedings.[23]

Defended by conservatives as opportunities for real people to make their voices heard and share their "wisdom," most observers believed that these kinds of activities were way over the line. As Ruth Conniff, journalist with *The Progressive* noted: "Clearly, the shout-downs at town halls are not a measure of public antipathy to health care reform. They are the product of political organizing. And that organizing is cynical, deceptive, and funded by special interests."[24] Table 4.1 shows how distorted the vocabulary of health care reform had become,[25] and Figure 4.1 captures these efforts as the Great Noise Machine of the right.[26]

TABLE 4.1

The Vocabulary of Health Care

WHAT IS SAID	WHAT IS HEARD
Universal health care	Socialized medicine
Health reform	Washington takeover
Individual mandate	Coerced health insurance
Shared responsibility	Higher taxes
Comparative effectiveness	Rationing of health care research
Public option	Predatory gov't, unfair competition
Advanced directives	Death panels
Health care exchange	Restricted choice
Medicare savings	Curtailed benefits, higher premiums
Rising numbers of uninsured	More "young invincibles"

Source: Wolfe, S. (Ed). Health debate or health charade? *Health Letter* 25 (10): 11, October, 2009.

FIGURE 4.1

The Great Noise Machine

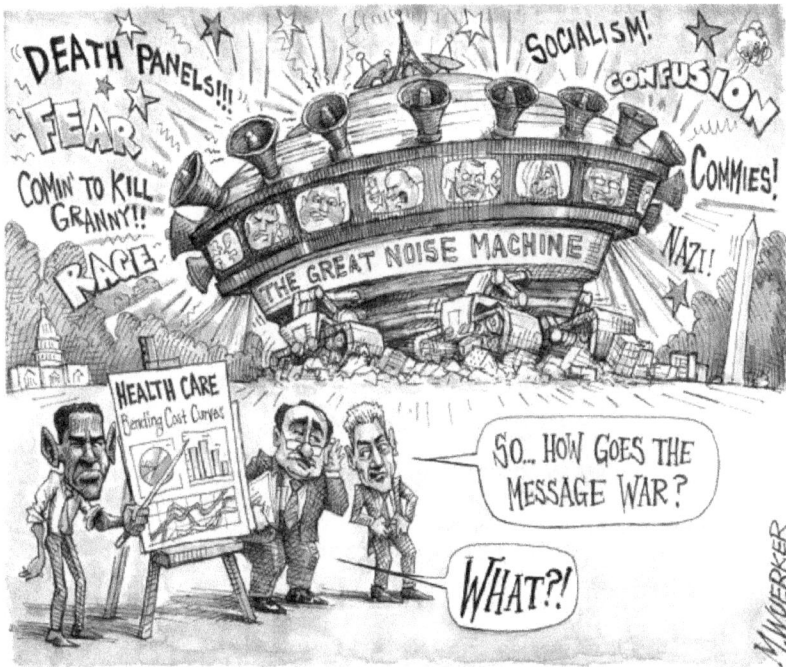

Source: Reprinted with permission of Matt Wuerker.

IMPACT OF PR CAMPAIGNS ON PUBLIC OPINION

By the middle of the Congressional recess in August, it appeared that the multi-media onslaught was having an effect among Americans in casting serious doubts about health reform bills in Congress. Although a majority of Americans have favored universal coverage through a government-guaranteed insurance system for everyone for many years (including 58 percent of respondents to a 2009 Kaiser Family Foundation survey),[27] raucous town hall meetings were surprisingly tolerated by many Americans. Independents were especially susceptible to changing their views on reform—two-thirds of Independent voters became more sympathetic to the protestors against reform. A *USA Today*/Gallup poll showed how respondents to a national survey viewed disruptive tactics, whether democracy in action or an abuse thereof (Figure 4.2).[28]

FIGURE 4.2

Town Hall Forums on Health Care: Abuse of Democracy?

Are the following actions at town-hall-style forums on health care
an example of democracy in action, or of the abuse of democracy?

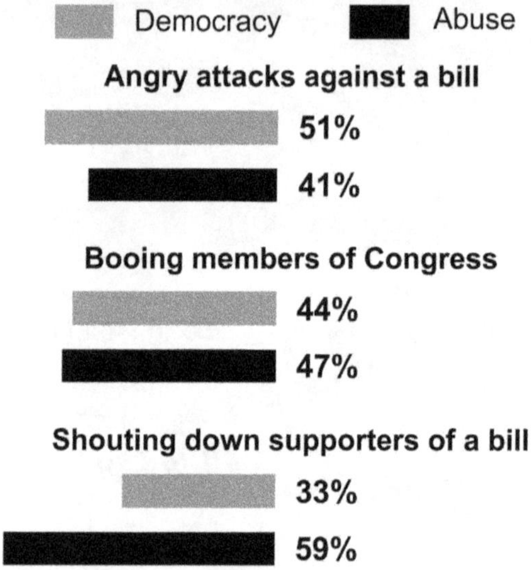

■ Democracy   ■ Abuse

Angry attacks against a bill

51%

41%

Booing members of Congress

44%

47%

Shouting down supporters of a bill

33%

59%

Source: Page, S. Protests tilt views on health care bill. *USA Today*, August 13, 2009.

The media blitz by conservative forces seeking to derail health care
reform and preserve our profit-driven multi-payer market-based system
involved all types of national media, including newspapers, television
and talk radio. False messages ranged from characterizing the legislation as the threat of "socialized medicine" to the beginning of rationed
care, from euthanasia for the elderly to the loss of choice or benefits
and intrusion by the government into the doctor-patient relationship.

By the end of the Congressional recess in August 2009, many
Americans were confused and uninformed on the issues. A CBS News
poll found that two-thirds of respondents found reform ideas too confusing to understand, while a CNN poll found that three in four Americans either wanted major changes to current health care bills, to abandon those bills and start over, or to stop all attempts at reform. A survey
by the Pew Center reported that Congressional favorability had fallen
to a 24-year low.[29]

We were all confused by the details of the changing health care bills as they worked their way through Congress, and as key provisions changed day by day. Even policy experts and journalists found it daunting to keep up with them, so it is not surprising that many voters were confused or uninformed on many details.

Over the 15-month period of the debate over health care reform ending in final votes on legislation in March 2010, Americans became deeply split over bills working their way through Congress. A Kaiser Health Tracking Poll found nearly as many Americans felt that they would be worse off if legislation passed compared to those who believed they would be better off (Figure 4.3). Support and opposition to these bills were sharply divided along party lines—support vs. oppose 75

FIGURE 4.3

Impact of Health Care Reform On Own Family

Do you think you and your family would be better or worse off if the president and Congress passed health care reform, or don't you think it would make much difference?

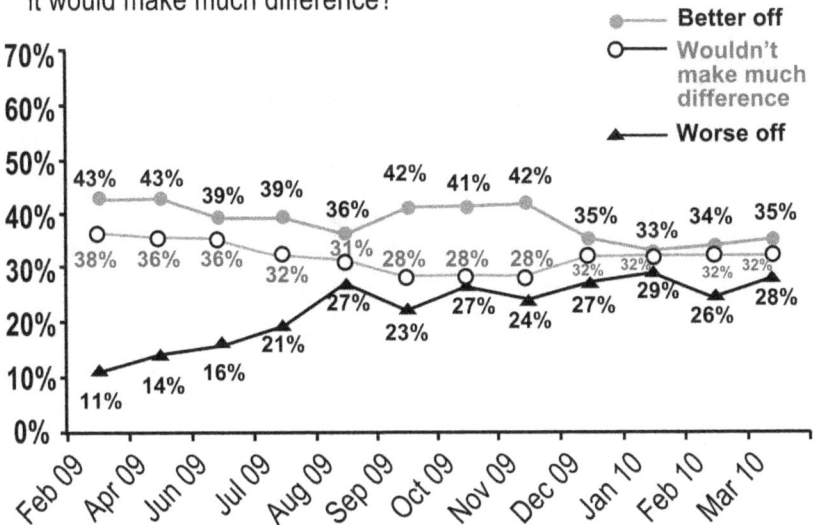

Source: Kaiser Health Tracking poll—March 2010 – Chartpack (#8058-C), The Henry J. Kaiser Foundation, March 2010. This information was reprinted with permission from the Henry J. Kaiser Foundation. The Kaiser Family Foundation is a non-profit private operating foundation, based in Menlo Park, California, dedicated to producing and communicating the best possible analysis and information on health issues.

percent vs. 15 percent for Democrats, 13 percent vs. 80 percent for Republicans, and 36 percent vs. 48 percent among Independents.[30]

We can ask how big a factor these distorted PR campaigns were in influencing public opinion toward health care reform. Based on what we saw in chapter 2, I would argue that corporate lobbying and campaign donations to politicians on the take played a much larger role than PR efforts in shaping the final outcome of legislation. There is no evidence in the health care debate that showed any erosion in long-standing broad support for single payer. Instead, we saw continued strong majority support for the public option, diminished as it became over the course of the campaign. As we will see in Chapter 7, when the public option was finally killed, it was not because of loss of public support but because Senator Joe Lieberman from Connecticut (the Senator from Aetna) threatened to filibuster against it in the Senate. In Connecticut, 84 percent of voters disapproved of his handling of the issue, even including 52 percent of *non-supporters* of the Senate bill.[31]

While it is not possible to ferret out the precise impact of these PR campaigns on public opinion amidst the swirling debate over complex issues, the three D's probably played some role in influencing the electorate. It is likely, however, that much of the public did see through the smoke and mirrors of 3-D rhetoric by both parties.

Sequential *Wall Street Journal*/NBC polls from September 2009 to March 2010 revealed the reasons that respondents either supported or opposed the legislation (Figure 4.4).[32] The public *did* get the essential points of reform alternatives. For example, even among supporters of the bills, only one in five respondents believed that they would lower or control health care costs (in spite of the hype by most Democrats) while the same small minority worried about Medicare cuts (again reflecting skepticism of fear-mongering by Republicans). Meanwhile, seven of ten Americans, across party lines, agreed that the policymaking process for health care reform was broken, certainly an accurate perception as this book documents.[33]

WHY THE DISTORTED DEBATE MATTERS

In short, distortions matter because they helped to derail health care reform completely from its initial objectives—containing health care costs and gaining universal access to affordable care of better quality. The slippery slope away from these goals has been remarkable, though

FIGURE 4.4

Divided on Health Care: Opponents point to cost, supporters cite expanded coverage

IS PRESIDENT OBAMA'S HEALTH-CARE PLAN A GOOD IDEA OR A BAD IDEA?

	Sept. 2009	Oct.	Dec.	Mar. 2010
Bad Idea	41%	42%	47%	48%
Not Sure	20%	20%	21%	16%
Good idea	39%	38%	32%	36%

WOULD IT BE BETTER TO PASS THE PLAN OR KEEP THE CURRENT SYSTEM?

	Sept. 2009	Oct.	Dec.	Mar. 2010
Keep Current System	39%	39%	44%	45%
Not Sure	16%	20%	15%	9%
Pass this Plan	45%	45%	41%	46%

REASONS FOR OPPOSING THE HEALTH-CARE LEGISLATION
among those who think it is a bad idea (up to two answers possible)

Too big, tries to change too many things at once	40%
Could increase the federal deficit	31%
Could raise taxes	31%
Could expand the role of government in providing health care	29%
Could cut funding to Medicare	26%

REASONS FOR SUPPORTING THE HEALTH-CARE LEGISLATION
among those who think it is a good idea

Could provide coverage for almost all Americans	45%
Allows people to get and keep insurance even with a pre-existing condition	38%
Could prevent insurance companies from unfairly raising premiums	32%
Could help lower, control costs	24%
Could be years before there is another chance to fix health care	11%

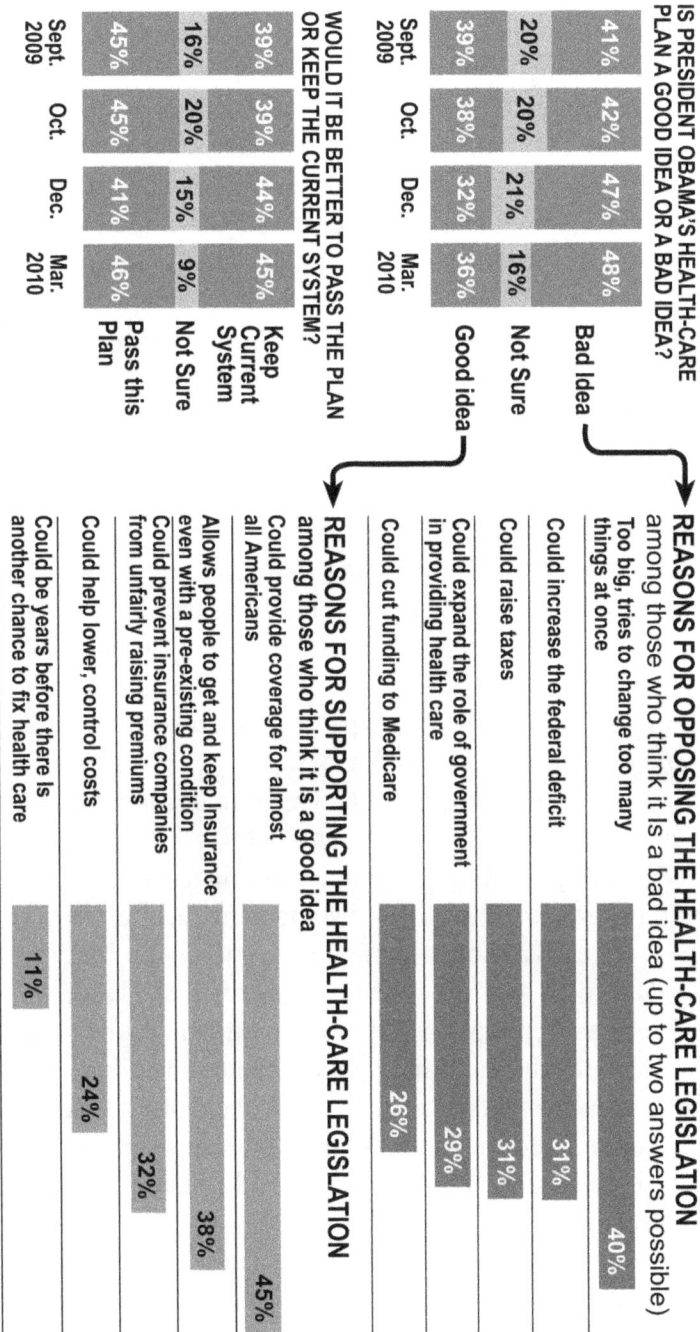

Source: Reprinted with permission from Wallsten, P, Spencer, J. Overhaul splits party faithful. *Wall Street Journal*, March 17, 2010: A8.

entirely predictable.

Fear mongering, orchestrated by corporate stakeholders and their surrogates, played a role in disconnecting the political discourse from reality and fomenting opposition to reform. This tactic has a long history in American politics. Jonathan Oberlander, political scientist at the University of North Carolina, reminds us that opposition to national health insurance around 1915 was fomented by claims that it was a plot by the German emperor to take over the United States. In the later 1940s, when national health insurance was again proposed, the AMA led a scare campaign that it would lead to Communism, with the Red army marching on our streets. Fast forward to our times today—as Oberlander observes: "Fear is crowding out the truth. And the truth ought to count for something in health care reform and American politics. And right now it doesn't."[34]

Unfortunately, as we saw in the last chapter, a flawed frame was used to define the options for health care reform. Special interests and their allies were successful in imposing their frames of policy alternatives as a means of exploiting health care to their advantage. They do this very well. Single payer was never on the table. The insurance industry's pledge (Chapter 1) looked like reform and seduced many liberals and policy makers into thinking that a bipartisan approach to a multi-payer system could remedy our cost and access problems. That left a weak public option as the maximal insurance reform, destined to fail due to its many restrictions and lack of market clout.

We need to recognize the gaping disconnect in the logic and behavior of the health insurance industry. As discussed in detail elsewhere,[35] the industry has proven itself over many decades to be too inefficient and too self-serving to be worthy of the public trust. Its pledge of partial "reforms," such as elimination of pre-existing conditions as a reason for non-issue in exchange for a government-subsidized individual mandate, was a Faustian bargain extending their profits well into the future by derailing reform. Even as small and impotent as the public option became, AHIP fought hard to kill it as the feared "stalking horse for single payer."

Democracy failed us throughout this latest health care reform attempt, arguably the most important domestic issue affecting us all. Our political process has been corrupted by special interests protecting their turfs and profits, as has happened so many times in the past. The town hall mobs, attended by howling, sometimes armed protestors recruited by special interests opposed to reform, make a mockery of our claimed democratic process. True to form, the health care debate was hijacked by corporate stakeholder cash generated from profits off *our* money—what we will pay on uncontrolled prices and on taxes for a failing system.

As is clear from these four opening chapters, real health care reform faces powerful enemies who can buy Congress, frame debates, and deploy massive resources in an effort to influence the public. That leads us to ask: who is standing up for the public interest—President Obama? The Democrats? The next three chapters will answer that question, as we turn next to the role of the corporate media in this battle.

References

1. Weisman, J, King, N, Adamy, J. Wrong turns: How Obama's health-care push went astray. *Wall Street Journal*, September 3. 2009: A4.
2. Sullivan, K. Americans support single payer. Why doesn't Celinda Lake? Blog posting, December 11, 2008 on PNHP web site.
3. Obama, B. Presidential address to the Democratic caucus in the House. Washington, D.C., March 20, 2010.
4. Hightower, J. Taking us for a ride on health care 'reform'. *The Progressive Populist* 15 (16), September 15, 2009: p 3.
5. Web site for Conservatives for Patients' Rights, accessed October 5, 2009.
6. Mullins, B, Kilman, S. Lobbyists line up to torpedo speech proposals. *Wall Street Journal*, February 26, 2009: A4.
7. Web site for FreedomWorks, accessed October 5 2009.
8. Ibid # 2.
9. Arnst, C. The best medical care in the U.S. *Business Week*, July 17, 2006.
10. Kerr, EA, Gerzoff, RB, Krein, SL, Selby, JV, Piette, JD et al. Diabetes care quality in the Veterans Administration Health Care System and commercial managed care: The TRIAD study. *Ann Intern Med* 141 (4): 272-81, 2004.
11. Peterson, LA, Normand, SL, Leape, LL, McNeil, BJ. Comparison of use of medications after acute myocardial infarction in the Veterans Health Administration and Medicare. *Circulation* 104 (24): 2898-904, 2001.
12. Web site for Americans for Prosperity, accessed October 5, 2009.
13. Zweifel, D. Brain tumor ad just propaganda. *The Progressive Populist* 15 (15), September 1, 2009, p 7.
14. Potter, W. Rally against Wall Street's health care takeover. *Truthout*, September 1, 2009.
15. Web site of Club for Growth, accessed October 5, 2009.
16. Bendavid, N. Scare tactics cast government, insurers in role of villains. *Wall*

Street Journal, August 10, 2009: A4.

17. Web site for Council for affordable health insurance, accessed October 5, 2009.

18. Reinhardt, UE. What portion of premiums should insurers pay out in benefits? *New York Times*, October 2, 2009.

19. Web site of Americans for Stable Quality Care, accessed October 5, 2009.

20. The ad campaign. Americans for Stable Quality Care. *New York Times* on line, August 15, 2009.

21. Krugman, P. The town hall mob. *New York Times*, August 7, 2009: A 17.

22. Collins, G. Gunning for health care. *New York Times,* August 13, 2009: A 21.

23. Herszenhorn, DM, Stolbert, SG. Health plan opponents make their voices heard. *New York Times*, August 4, 2009: A 12.

24. Cunniff, R. Losing the health care shouting match. *The Progressive*, August 10, 2009.

25. Wolf, S (Ed). Health debate or health charade? *Health Letter* 25 (10): 11, October, 2009.

26. Baker, D. The public plan option and the big government conservatives. *The Progressive Populist* 15:18, October 15, 2009: p 12.

27. Thomas, H. Health care for all. Politics blog, August 13, 2009.

28. Page, S. Protests tilt views on health care bill. *USA Today*, August 13, 2009.

29. Blow, C. The prince of dispassion. Op-Ed. *New York Times*, September 5, 2009: A15.

30. Kaiser Health Tracking Poll, March 2010. Kaiser Family Foundation. Publication Number 8058, March 19, 2010.

31. TalkingPointsMemo (http://tpmdc.talkingpointsmemo.com/2010/01/poll-lieberman-hated-by-everyone-in-connecticut-after-health-care-debates.php.

32. Wallsten, P, Spencer,J. Overhaul splits party faithful. *Wall Street Journal*, March 17, 2010: A8.

33. Ibid # 31.

34. Rovner, J. In health care debate, fear trumps logic. *NPR,* August 28, 2009.

35. Geyman, JP. *Do Not Resuscitate: Why the Health Insurance Industry Is Dying, and How We Must Replace It.* Monroe, ME. Common Courage Press, 2009.

CHAPTER 5

Media and Money:
Broadcasting Corporate Values

"A popular government without popular information or the means of acquiring it is but a Prologue to a Farce or a Tragedy or perhaps both."
— James Madison, one of our Founding Fathers and fourth president of the United States[1]

President James Madison's concern some two centuries ago shows that the impact of corrupted news on our democracy is an age-old problem. That leads us to ask how this problem plays out today, especially with regard to the politics of health care reform.

Today, independent, objective and reliable news is becoming more the exception than the rule. The corporate reach of commercial "journalism" now extends to all forms of media, including print, digital, television and radio. Investigative journalism is declining for lack of funding as corporate media owners downsize editorial and reporting staffs. Newspapers are collapsing all over the country; the Internet has become a major information source for a growing part of the population despite its variable standards of accuracy or accountability; media conglomerates with deep pockets lobby for policies allowing even more mergers to gain monopoly positions; and incisive reporting on the activities of government at all levels—from city halls to state and federal levels—is on the decline.[2] All of these trends increase the ability of corporate media to offer "information" masquerading as news, serving their own needs more than the public interest. As Robert McChesney and John Nichols observe in their excellent book, *The Death and Life of American Journalism: The Media Revolution that Will Begin the World Again*:

"This is not a routine crisis. It fundamentally brings to a head the long-simmering tension between journalism and commerce."[3]

This chapter will examine this relationship of the media to health care reform by addressing two questions: (1) How do the corporate media distort the real issues and manipulate "information" biased toward corporate interests? and (2) What are the implications of their failure to report accurately on the big issues?

CORPORATE MEDIA—
BOUGHT AND PAID FOR BY INDUSTRY

These are some of the major ways in which corporate interests drive the debate over health care reform:

Corporate Media Catering to Industry

Katharine Weymouth, publisher of the *Washington Post*, was a CEO with a plan. In mid-summer 2009 it was time for her paper to get into the act and raise some cash off the health care reform efforts. Uncovered by the web site *Politico*, Weymouth schemed to host a dozen off-the-record "salons" at her Washington, D.C. home, convening lobbyists, politicians, invited members from the Administration, and some of her editors and reporters for discussions of health care policy. Each event was be underwritten by major players in select policy areas. The first, titled *Healthcare Reform: Better or Worse for Americans*? was to be sponsored by Kaiser Permanente.[4]

Invitees were to buy their way to the table for these private dinner parties, each with a maximal attendance of 20 people. The *Post* offered them sponsorship of individual salons for $25,000 (maximum of two sponsors per salon), or an annual series sponsorship of 11 salons for $250,000. A promotional flyer offered:

> "An exclusive opportunity to participate in the health-care re-form debate among the select few who will actually get it done...
> A unique opportunity for stakeholders to hear and be heard...
> At the core is a critical topic of our day... By bringing togeth-er those powerful few in business and policy-making who are forwarding, legislating and reporting on the issues, Washington Post Salons give life to the debate. Be at this nexus of business and policy with your underwriting of Washington Post Salons."[5]

Revelation of this plan created a firestorm of protest and was a public relations disaster for the *Washington Post*. Weymouth (also an attorney and graduate of the Harvard School of Business) hastily cancelled all plans for these salons, giving a limp explanation that the flyer had been produced by the paper's marketing department, had not been vetted by her or the newsroom, and "completely misrepresented what we were trying to do." Other reporters, however, soon learned that some of the invitations had been sent from Weymouth's personal email, and that Marcus Brauchli, the Executive Editor, was aware of the salons and planned to attend, though he said that he "did not understand exactly what the party was."[6] Faced by an uproar among *Post* reporters, he immediately issued an email to the newsroom labeled *Newsroom Independence*:

> "Colleagues, a flyer was distributed this week offering an 'underwriting opportunity' for a dinner on health care reform, in which the news department had been asked to participate. The language in the flyer and the description of the event preclude our participation."[7]

Unfortunately, such cozy relationships between stakeholders and the media are common, though this example was more brazen than most in selling opportunities to spin the news in the interests of sponsoring stakeholders. Similar arrangements have been made by other publications, including the *Wall Street Journal*, *Newsweek*, the *Los Angeles Times*, and the *Atlantic*. Even *Politico,* which ironically was started by two ex-*Washington Post* reporters, has sponsored similar events, such as a party at the 2008 Democratic National Convention with a large Washington D.C.-based lobbying firm, the Glover Park Group. Figure 5.1, from the cover of the September 2009 issue of *Extra!*, the publication of the media watchdog group Fairness and Accuracy in Reporting (FAIR), illustrates these ethical problems. And Peter Hart, Director of Activism at FAIR observed:

> "News outlets trying to defend such practices sound like politicians who claim to be unaffected by the lobbyists and deep-pocketed contributors who bankroll their political careers. Such hollow claims of independence are dismissed by most observers of American politics. There is no reason to judge news outlets by a different standard."[8]

FIGURE 5.1

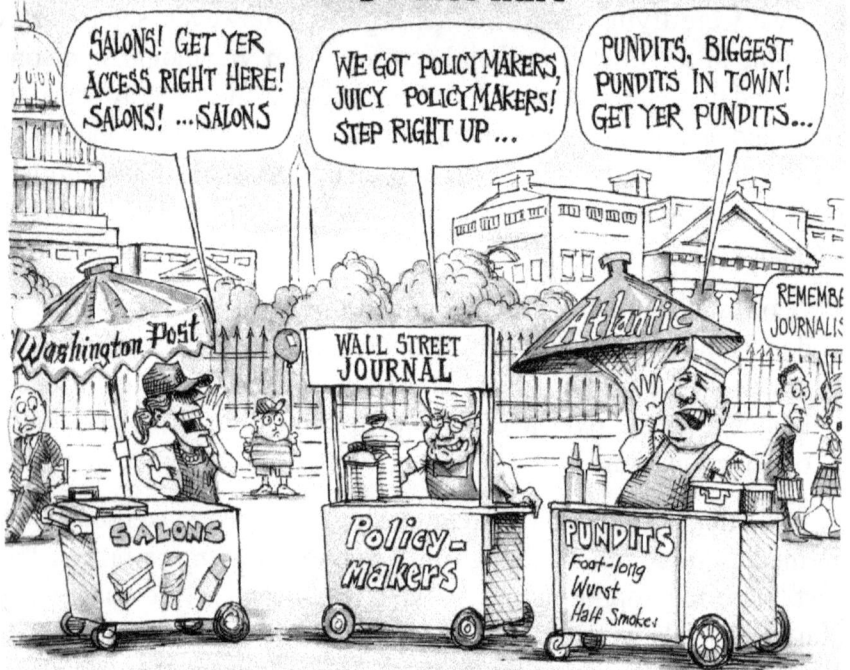

Source: Reprinted with permission of Matt Wuerker from Hart, P. Journalistic reputations for sale. *Extra!* 22 (9), September 2009.

In addition to the conflict-of-interest relationships described above, there is an ongoing media-lobbying complex not apparent to the general public. A recent four-month investigation by *The Nation* found that at least 75 registered lobbyists, public relations representatives and corporate officials have appeared since 2007 on MSNBC, Fox News, CNN, CNBC and Fox Business Network without disclosure of their corporate financial ties.

When Richard Gephardt declared on MSNBC's *Morning Meeting* that the public option is not essential, there was no mention of the work his lobbying firm Gephardt Government Affairs was doing for the insurance industry or that he was a paid lobbyist for NBC/Universal.

As Janine Wedel of George Washington University's School of Public Policy observed:

> "While these influence peddlers are not necessarily unethical, they elude accountability to governments, shareholders and voters—and threaten democracy. When there's a whole host of pundits on the airwaves touting the same agenda at the same time, you get a cumulative effect that shapes public opinion toward their agenda."[9]

Ties to Conservative Talk Shows, Writers and Editors

Rupert Murdoch is one of the biggest media power brokers in the world. A glimpse into his activities to influence and control political discourse gives an idea how extensive is the reach of a media mogul.

Murdoch developed a number of publications in his native Australia before expanding his News Corporation (News Corp) into the United Kingdom, where he diversified into television by creating Sky Television in 1989. He soon became known for his sharp business practices, persistent interference with his editors, and a tendency toward tabloid sensationalism. He became an American citizen in 1987, which allowed him to own American television stations. By the mid-1990s, Murdoch owned Fox Network, established the 24-hour cable news station Fox News Channel, and launched the conservative *The Weekly Standard*. In a battle with CNN for market share, he soon proclaimed Fox News as "the most-watched cable news channel." In the late 1990s, he expanded his media empire into Asia. Since the turn of this century, he has become a leading investor in satellite television, the film industry and the Internet. In 2007, he bought Dow Jones, owner of the *Wall Street Journal*. According to the 2009 Forbes 44, he had a net worth of about $4 billion and was the 132nd richest person in the world.[10]

If one wonders about editorial independence on major political issues of the day, the buildup to the 2003 invasion of Iraq gives us the answer. All 175 of Murdoch owned newspapers editorialized in favor of the war.[11]

The editorial policies of the *Wall Street Journal,* as with other of Murdoch's news outlets, have been clearly stated in many ways concerning the economy, health care and the roles of the market vs.

government. They consistently advocate for free markets with minimal government regulation. Concerning health care reform, they argue against price controls and for the freedom of people to "choose" the kind of care they need, with little regard for whether they can actually afford necessary care.

Murdoch's hiring of Glenn Beck to host a Fox News program shows us how effectively he can manipulate the "news" and drum up support for his own agenda. He tasked Beck to put together The 9-12 Project with the goal to "bring America back to where it was on September 12, 2001," the day after the terrorist attacks. This project's website serves as a social-networking device promoting right wing views, nationalism, and fears about the direction of the country. In the effort to derail health care reform, it has been credited with helping to organize disrupters of town hall meetings during the August 2009 congressional recess. Together with other right-wing organizations, such as TeaPartyExpress.org and Our Country Deserves Better PAC, it helped to promote the march on Washington, D.C. on September 12, 2009.[12]

Eric Alterman, Distinguished Professor of English and Journalism at Brooklyn College and Professor of Journalism at the CUNY Graduate School of Journalism, describes Fox as a propaganda outlet, and an extremist one at that. In making this case, he asks whether a genuine news organization would, as Fox has done:

- "run, over a five-day period, twenty-two excerpts from healthcare forums in which every single speaker was opposed?
- allow a producer to cheer-lead, off camera, anti-Obama pro-testers?
- run these kinds of headlines, as a 'Fox Nation Victory': SENATE REMOVES 'END OF LIFE' PROVISION and CONGRESS DELAYS HEALTH CARE RATIONING BILL?"[13]

Murdoch's media empire extends to book publishers as well. His HarperCollins publishes conservative-oriented books, such as those by Peggy Noonan, former Reagan speech writer and *Wall Street Journal* columnist.[14]

Interlocking Directorates
Interlocking directorates, whereby directors of one corporation

sit on one or more other corporate boards, is more the rule than the exception. This creates an obvious conflict of interest when the missions or policies of companies differ. And when media companies are involved, the conflicts are increased further when editors and journalists are called upon to deal with stories that would likely involve a loss of revenue to their employers.

A recent study by FAIR revealed how extensive these inter-connections are. Among nine major media corporations and their major outlets—Disney (ABC), General Electric (NBC), CBS, Time Warner (CNN, *Time*), News Corporation (Fox), New York Times Co., Washington Post Co. (*Newsweek*), Tribune Co. (*Chicago Tribune, Los Angeles Times*) and Gannett (*USA Today*)—there were connections to six different insurance companies. Two insurance companies—Chubb and Berkshire Hathaway—had more than one media corporation director. Six of the nine media corporations had board connections with pharmaceutical companies. Table 5.1 lists the interlocking directorates

TABLE 5.1

Interlocking Directorates

Media Corporation	Insurance & Pharmaceutical Companies
Disney (ABC)	Proctor & Gamble
GE (NBC)	Chubb, Novartis, Proctor & Gamble, Merck
Time Warner (CNN)	AIG, Health Cap, Paratek Pharmaceuticals
Fox/News Corp.	GlaxoSmithKline, Genentech Hybritech
New York Times Co.	First Health Group, Eli Lilly
Washington Post/Newsweek	Berkshire Hathaway, Markel
Tribune Co.	Abbott Labs, Middlebrook Pharmaceuticals
Gannett/Ms Today	Chubb

Source: Murphy, K. Single payer & interlocking directorates. *Extra!*, August 2009, p 7.

of these nine media corporations.[15]

Although single payer national health insurance has been favored by a majority of Americans for some 40 years and would effectively address the country's crisis in access to affordable health care for everyone, it was barely covered by the U.S. media. Out of many thousands of reports on health care reform in the first six months of 2009, for example, single payer was mentioned in only 164 articles or news segments. More than 70 percent of those mentions did not include input from a single payer advocate. Among the few that did include a single payer voice, most were accounted for by a single program—the *Ed Show* on MSNBC. We can only conclude from this media coverage that the interests of the insurance and drug industries are fundamentally aligned.[16]

Advertising on Local TV

The health care reform debate is just what the doctor ordered for local television stations, beleaguered as they are in the economic downturn. As they have tried to cope with sharp declines in advertising revenue, the late spring and early summer of 2009 found them taking in about $1 million a day in ads on health care related subjects. The Campaign Media Analysis Group at TNS, a research firm owned by ad holding company WPP, reported that some $41 million had been spent on local TV spots by July, mostly in the last few weeks of that period. The group estimated that ad revenue might reach $250 million for the year, since a prolonged debate would "open the door even wider for opponents to appeal to the public." At that time, most of the ad spending on health care was being spent for local TV stations and national cable news networks such as News Corp's Fox News and Time Warner's CNN.[17]

Lobbying groups were targeting their TV ads to areas where legislators were pivotal to the outcome of health care reform legislation. The content of ads were on both sides of the reform issue. But among the most widely aired was the ad created by the Americans for Prosperity Foundation featuring the false claim, as mentioned in the previous chapter, that a Canadian woman with a "brain tumor" would have died in Canada had she not sought immediate care in the U.S. Other ads were placed on narrower issues, such as those by PhRMA on the role of biotech companies in working to cure Alzheimer's disease and diabetes.[18]

Feeding Talking Points to Media

In her excellent article on how right-wing operatives play the "inside-outside" game, journalist Adele Stan tells us how some of these operatives have served the right since the 1960s. Richard Viguerie helped get Ronald Reagan elected in 1980 by harnessing the power of direct-mail solicitations. The late Paul Weyrich founded the Heritage Foundation, which then became a spin and policy factory for the Reagan Administration. Howard Phillips focused on the outside game, organizing angry citizens and even founding his own political party, the U.S. Taxpayer Party (now the Constitution Party). Through his Conservative Caucus, Phillips has long railed against the danger of "socialized medicine," has argued that Medicare is unconstitutional, has referred to Planned Parenthood as "Murder Incorporated," has warned against euthanasia by the government, and more recently, has spread the "birther" theory that President Obama is not an American citizen.[19]

Betsy McCaughey gives us another example of how lies and distortions are promulgated as "news". During the 1993-1994 effort to enact the Clinton Health Plan, she worked off-the-record with the tobacco industry to derail that program, which would have been partly funded by large increases in taxes on tobacco.[20] As an economist with the National Center for Policy Analysis (NCPA), a well-funded conservative Dallas-based think tank, she promulgated the idea that the U.S. health care system is the best in the world, partly basing this claim on better five-year survival statistics compared to other advanced countries.[21] I have rebutted that claim and the use of that particular quality measure in a recent book, *The Cancer Generation: Baby Boomers Facing a Perfect Storm*. There is abundant evidence that we do *not* have the best medical care in the world.[22] This time around, she incited the opposition to health care reform by inventing the term "death panels" and warning that we would have to deal with them under the Obama plan.[23]

HEALTH CARE REFORM AND MEDIA FAILURE

The corporate media have failed miserably to educate the public on the real issues of health care reform. Reporters of the major media tend to explain this as a result of the complexity of the health care system.

John Harwood of the *New York Times* notes that health care issues are neither cable TV-friendly nor journalism-friendly stories. Julie Rovner of *NPR* recently told *Politico* that "the problem with health care is that it's so big and so complicated that the public is never really going to understand all the moving parts of this."[24]

But as we have seen in the last two chapters, there is much more to the story of why the media have yet to cover health care well. As Peter Hart of FAIR observes:

> "It was probably a given that the corporate press would mangle the debate over this year's healthcare reform legislation, considering their poor showing in the healthcare debate of the early '90s. The only questions were when and how. One answer came immediately, as the media shut off discussion of a popular single payer plan before it even started. But in the debate the media did allow, the answer came in late summer when "town hall" protests and the media's fetish for bipartisanship pushed the discourse well to the right."[25]

All this is not new. A hundred years ago, muckraking journalists reported that large corporations and other wealthy interests used bribery, fraud and even blackmail to dominate politics and get their way. As virtual owners of the country, jokes were often made about "the Senator from Standard Oil." One courageous reporter—David Graham Phillips—wrote this in the March 1906 issue of *Cosmopolitan Magazine*, as in the first of nine articles under the title *"The Treason of the Senate:"*

> "Treason is a strong word, but not too strong, rather too weak, to characterize the situation in which the Senate is the eager, resourceful, indefatigable agent of interests as hostile to the American people as any invading army could be, and vastly more dangerous: interests that manipulate the prosperity produced by all, so that it heaps up riches for the few: interests whose growth and power can only mean the degradation of the people, of the educated into sycophants, of the masses toward serfdom."[26]

Phillips and other muckraking journalists provoked such public outrage that the 17th amendment was added to the Constitution providing for the direct popular election of senators instead of the previous system whereby they were elected by state legislators who were easily bought off.[27]

Fast forward to the end of the 1990s, when James Carey, professor of journalism at Columbia University, had this to say about the status of journalism:

"We have a journalism that reports the continuing stream of expert opinion, but because there is not agreement among experts, it is more like observing talk-show gossip and petty manipulation than bearing witness to the truth. We have a journalism of fact without regard to understanding through which the public is immobilized and demobilized and merely ratifies the judgments of experts delivered from on high. It is above all a journalism that justifies itself in the public's name but in which the public plays no role except as an audience: a receptacle to be informed by experts and an excuse for the practice of publicity."[28]

Trudy Lieberman, Director of the Health and Medicine Reporting Program at the City University of New York's Graduate School of Journalism, gives us this further observation:

"The right wing's mastery of publicity, and its success in shutting out other points of view and turning major issues affecting millions of people into lopsided discourse, shows this kind of journalism is just not good enough."[29]

In his landmark book *Moyers On Democracy*, Bill Moyers brings us this important observation:

"'Limited government' has little to do anymore with the Constitution or local autonomy; now it means corporate domination and the shifting of risk from government and business to struggling families and workers. 'Family values' now means imposing a sectarian definition on everyone else. 'Religious freedom' means majoritarianism and public benefits for organized religion without any public burdens. And 'patriotism' means blind support for failed leaders. It's what happens when an interlocking media system filters through commercial values and ideology the information and moral viewpoints that people consume in their daily lives."[30]

Can the many abuses of the public interest with which the

corporate media are a complicit partner stir enough public outrage today to advance much needed reforms of health care? The aftermath of courageous reporting by a few journalists a century ago give us hope that an emboldened media rededicated to ethical standards of the journalism profession can bring about such positive change. But today's challenges to rebuild a corrupted media in the public interest will be a heavy lift. McChesney and Nichols urge us to borrow from the experience and wisdom of other countries, such as the United Kingdom, Japan, Denmark and other European countries that invest in serious public interest journalism (Figure 5.2).[31] They leave us this challenge:

> "The old order is collapsing, brought down by its own compromises and corruptions. There will be a new order, but it need not be a reflection of that which caused the crisis. We can grab what is good and necessary from the crumbling edifice—serious journalism, with its scope, skepticism and strength—and raise it up on a new platform that is freer, faster and fiercer in its determination to

FIGURE 5.2

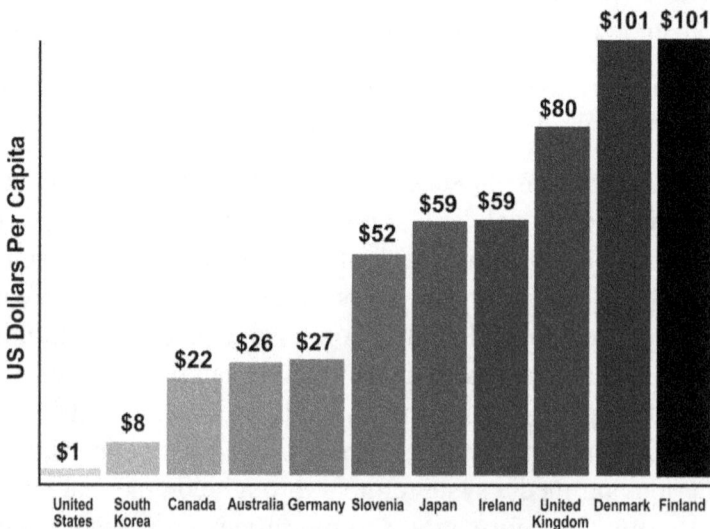

Global Spending on Public Media, 2007

Source: Reprinted with permission from McChesney, RW, Nichols, J. *The Death and Life of American Journalism*. Philadelphia. Nation Books, 2010, p 274.

communicate the whole story to all the people."[32]

References

1. Madison, J. As quoted in McChesney, RW, Nichols, J. *The Death and Life of American Journalism.* Philadelphia. Nation Books, 2010, p. 2.

2. Alterman, E. Money for nothing. *The Nation* 290 (12): 10, March 29, 2010.

3. McChesney, RW, Nichols, J. *The Death and Life of American Journalism.* Philadelphia. Nation Books, 2010, p.11.

4. Perez-Pena, R. Pay-for-chat plan falls flat at Washington Post. *New York Times,* July 3, 2009: A1.

5. Allen, M, Calderone, M. Washington Post cancels lobbyist event amid uproar. *Truthout,* July 2, 2009.

6. Carr, D. A publisher stumbles publicly at the Post. *New York Times,* July 4, 2009: B1.

7. Ibid # 5.

8. Hart, P. Journalistic reputations for sale. Extra! 22 (9): 7-8, September 2009.

9. Jones, S. The media-lobbying complex. *The Nation* 290 (8): 14, March 1, 2010.

10. Wikipedia, listing for Rupert Murdoch, accessed on October 17, 2009.

11. Ibid # 10.

12. Stan, AM. Inside story on town hall riots: Right-wing shock troops do corporate America's dirty work. *Alternet,* August 10. 2009.

13. Alterman, E. Just don't call it 'journalism". *The Nation* 289(15):10, November 9, 2009.

14. Ibid # 12.

15. Murphy, K. Single payer & interlocking directorates. Extra!, August 2009, p 7.

16. Ibid # 15.

17. Vranica, S, Mundy, A. Advertising. Health-care debate is tonic for local TV. *Wall Street Journal,* July 27, 2009: B5.

18. Ibid # 17.

19. Ibid # 12.

20. EIN News, 'Death panel' inventor has close ties to Philip Morris, September 21, 2009.

21. McCaughey, B. U.S. cancer care is number one. Brief Analysis No. 596. Dallas, TX. National Center for Policy Analysis, October 11, 2007.

22. Geyman, JP. *The Cancer Generation: Baby Boomers Facing a Perfect Storm.* Monroe, ME. Common Courage Press, 2009: pp34-6, 114-19.

23. EIN News. 'Death panel' inventor Betsy McCaughey has close ties to Philip Morris, September 21, 2009.

24. Hart, P. Healthcare reform minus the public option—or the public. Extra! 22:10, October, 2009, p 7.

25. Ibid # 24.

26. Moyers, B, Winship, M. In Washington, the revolving door is hazardous to your health. *Truthout,* October 11, 2009.

27. Ibid # 26.
28. Carey, J. *Journalists Just Leave: The Ethics of an Anomalous Profession,* in *The Media & Morality*, edited by Baird, RM, Loges, WE, and Rosenbaum, SE. Amherst, NY, Prometheus Books, 1999, p 51.
29. Lieberman, T. *Slanting the Story: The Forces That Shape the News*. New York. The New Press, 2000, p 167.
30. Moyers, B. *Moyers On Democracy.* New York. Anchor Books, 2008, p 319.
31. Ibid # 2, p 274.
32. Ibid # 2, pp 228-9.

CHAPTER 6

Missing in Action:
Public Opinion and the Public Interest

"The White House and Congress claimed throughout the [health care reform] process that we must retain private insurance because Americans desire choice of insurance, and this has been framed as choice of insurance. However, this is a false concept. No person can anticipate what their health care needs will be or which insurance will be best. Health care needs change the day a patient has a serious accident or is diagnosed with a serious illness. We all need the same health insurance: one that covers all medically necessary care when and where we need it."

—Margaret Flowers, M.D., pediatrician and Congressional Fellow for Physicians for a National Health Program, Washington, D.C.[1]

We saw in Chapter 3 how framing of health care reform issues *by both political parties* went way off track from the start of this latest effort to reform our system. Now, looking back at the entire political process, we have to ask who, if anyone, has stood up for the public interest? As we saw in the last chapter, certainly not the corporate media. So how about our newly elected leaders in Congress and the White House after the Democratic sweep of the 2008 elections?

This chapter has two goals: (1) to summarize public opinion in America over the last 60 years toward its health care system; and (2) to show how our political leadership turned away from popular will in making political compromises that place the interests of corporate stakeholders and their investors above the needs of ordinary Americans.

WHAT DOES THE PUBLIC WANT?
A BEDROCK OF SUPPORT FOR NHI

Support for a program of national health insurance in the U.S. goes back for more than six decades, despite what our politicians would like us to believe. That it is solid, consistent and unambiguous is indicated by the following time line of sequential surveys and studies:

- In the 1940s, 74 percent of the public supported such a plan.[2]
- In 1965, 61 percent of respondents supported Medicare, a single payer plan for people 65 years of age and older.[3]
- Between 1980 and 2000, public support for NHI in many polls ranged from 50 to 66 percent, when asked their opinion on a plan "financed by tax money, and paying for most forms of health care."[4] (Table 6.1)
- In 1997, a national survey by the National Coalition on Health Care found that four out of five respondents agreed that "medical care has become a big business that puts profits ahead of people" and three of five believed that the "federal government should play a more active role in assuring access to care."[5]
- A 1998 national survey reported that one-half of respondents believed that the federal government should guarantee access to care for all Americans, even if that required paying an additional tax of $2,000 a year.[6]
- In 2002, a national poll by Harris Interactive surveyed five different groups—citizens, physicians, employers, hospital managers, and health plan managers. One-half *in every group* favored radical reform of the health care system over incremental change.[7]
- In 2004, a study of 4,000 adults by the Commonwealth Fund found that 62 percent of Americans would be willing to forego the entire Bush tax cut in exchange for guaranteed health insurance for everyone.[8]
- In 2007, an Associated Press/Yahoo survey of more than 1,800 adults found that 65 percent of respondents believed that "the U.S. should adopt a universal health insurance program in which everyone is covered under a program like Medicare that is run by the government and financed by taxpayers;" that same year, two other major surveys by CNN/Opinion Research and

TABLE 6.1

Americans' Attitudes About National Health Insurance, 1980-2000

National Health Insurance, financed by tax money, and paying for most forms of health care*	Favor	Oppose	No Opinion
1980 (February)	50%	41%	9%
1980 (March)	46	43	11
1981	52	37	11
1990 (March-April)	56	34	10
1990 (October	64	27	8
1991 (June)	60	30	10
1991 (August)	54	33	12
1992 (January)	65	26	9
1992 (July)	66	25	9
1993 (January)	63	26	11
1993 (March)	59	29	12
1995	53	39	8
2000 (August)			
General public	56	32	12
Registered voters	54	34	12

*Sources: CBS News/*New York Times* polls (1980-95); Harvard School of Public Health/ICR poll (2000)
Source: Blendon, RJ, Benson, JM. Americans' views on health policy: A fifty-year historical perspective. *Health Affairs (Millwood)* 20 (2): 35, 2001.

the *New York Times*/CBS News also reported that two-thirds of respondents wanted the federal government to provide a national health insurance program for all Americans.[9]
- In 2008, a Harvard School of Public Health/Harris Interactive poll asked respondents whether they felt they would be better or worse off if we had "socialized medicine" in this country; despite using that provocative term, 45 percent believed they would be better off while 39 percent felt they would be worse off.[10]

- An analysis after the 2008 election by the Pew Research Center gives us another interesting perspective on public support for NHI, further debunking the idea that it is a radical, politically infeasible idea. Its studies have shown that the proportion of Americans who describe their political views as liberal, conservative or moderate over the last twenty years has remained remarkably stable. Today, 21 percent call themselves liberal, 38 percent conservative and 36 percent moderate. Figure 6.1 displays these differences by age group and party. But many conservatives, regardless of political affiliation, support the concept of NHI. The Pew Research Center's analysis found that conservatives were evenly split concerning a guarantee by the federal government of health insurance for all Americans, even if that involved increasing taxes.[11]

Even as opposition to health care reform grew in July 2009, a Zogby poll showed that the electorate was almost evenly divided on the basic structure of reform. Overall, a plurality of respondents agreed with

FIGURE 6.1

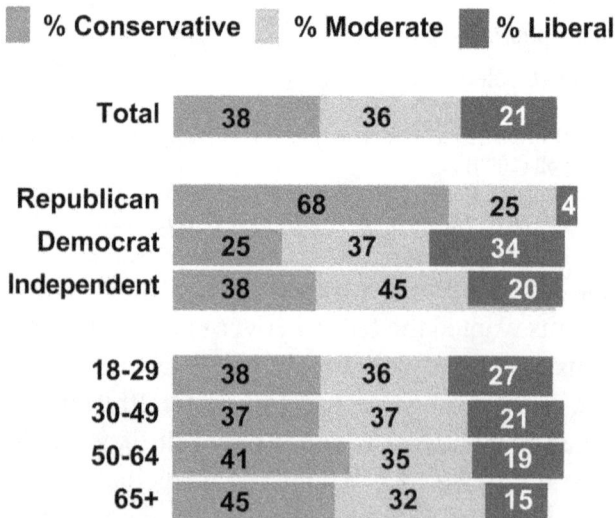

How Americans Describe Their Political Views

	% Conservative	% Moderate	% Liberal
Total	38	36	21
Republican	68	25	4
Democrat	25	37	34
Independent	38	45	20
18-29	38	36	27
30-49	37	37	21
50-64	41	35	19
65+	45	32	15

Source: Reprinted with permission from Horowitz, J. Winds of political change haven't shifted public's ideology balance. Pew Research Center Publications, November 28, 2009.

Plan A (a government-sponsored plan for universal health care) while Plan B (a single payer plan, Medicare for All) received slightly less support. More than four of five Democrats favored either Plan A or B (Table 6.2). Nine of ten Republicans opposed both with Independents leaning toward the Republicans' position.[12]

Do we need any more studies to know what Americans want in their health care system? Of course not! In fact, the disconnect of this well-documented public will and the outcome of the political process

TABLE 6.2

Public Support for Universal Plan A vs. Plan B

Plan A

Universal Plan A - " Do you agree or disagree with a universal health care plan that would require everyone in the U.S. to have health insurance with federal help for those who cannot pay the premiums?"

	Overall	Democrats	Independents	Republicans
Agree	49	86	43	11
Disagree	48	11	53	86
Not Sure	3	3	3	2

Plan B

Universal Plan B - " Do you agree or disagree with a universal health care plan where the government would provide health insurance for everyone in the U.S. under a single payer plan, similar to everyone having Medicare?"

	Overall	Democrats	Independents	Republicans
Agree	44	81	39	7
Disagree	52	15	57	91
Not Sure	4	5	4	2

Numbers may not add up to 100% due to rounding

In 2009, a plurality of residents (49%) agreed with Plan A, which most closely resembled the current reform proposals, while 48% disagreed. Plan B received slightly less support with only 44% agreeing to a potential "Medicare for all" system. The partisan split between Republicans and Democrats is significant.

Source: Zogby poll. American public remains divided over proposed health care reform. July 27, 2009.

over these last 60-plus years is remarkable. This majority consensus has been consistent over six decades, transcends political identity, has been unshakable despite an endless onslaught by defenders of our market-based system, politicians and the media, and has still been ignored by those in power regardless of their political party.

WHAT HAVE OUR POLITICAL LEADERS DONE THIS TIME?

As we can see, despite what conservatives and many moderates tell us about its "political infeasability," single payer NHI is hardly a fringe idea without widespread popular support. That single payer public financing of a private delivery system was never put on the table is a classic example of policymakers and politicians ignoring public opinion over many decades in this country. We could go so far as to call this legislative malpractice. The reasons for avoiding that option are obvious—it threatens revenue and profit streams of all members of the corporate medical industrial complex. Once again, their lobbyists and allies won the day in excluding single payer from the debate.

We have seen recurrent successful efforts over the years by opponents of single payer, led by stakeholders in our market-based system, to keep NHI in the closet. Two examples are especially disingenuous:

- In the 1990s, "citizen juries" were convened to debate whether or not the Clinton Health Plan was a good direction to pursue. Each was a 24-person jury of average Americans. After a five-day debate over a range of private and public options, the Clinton Health Plan, dubbed the "Health Insurance Preservation Act" by critics, was voted down, 19 to 5, while informal support was given to a single payer option, 17 to 7.[13]

- A Citizens' Health Care Working Group was established by the Medicare legislation of 2003 (MMA) to examine the problems of our health care system and make recommendations for approaches to address them. Over the next two years, many community meetings were held across the country. As a result, 96.8 percent of participants believed that our system was in crisis, while 94 percent believed that affordable health care should be a part of national health policy. Among ten policy alternatives toward that goal, single payer NHI was by far the leading reform option, supported by 46 percent of the 800 participants. Table 6.3

shows the overwhelming response to this option compared to the other nine alternatives.[14] These results, however, did not appear in the final recommendations of the Working Group submitted in 2006 for public review, which instead proposed a system of insurance policies for catastrophic illness with deductibles up to $30,000, an option that was not even discussed in community meetings and which triggered considerable opposition in online polls.[15]

The 2008 elections were a clear rejection of eight years of Republican leadership. Many believed that a major transformational change had taken place. The electorate had spoken, calling for new directions. So what happened to the change that we voted for, and would our newly elected leaders really act in the public's best interest?

Unfortunately, as we will see in following summary of events over the ensuing months, Obama and the Democrats were up to the same old tricks in paying no attention to the will of the public and distorting issues for their own political reasons.

The Baucus Eight incident gives us a good example of politicians' contempt for the will of the public during this last health care reform attempt. Senator Max Baucus (D-MT), as Chairman of the key Senate Finance Committee, played a pivotal role in how Congress dealt with reform legislation. We saw in Chapter 2 how beholden he has been to campaign contributions from health care industries over the years. His rejection of single payer was well-known. In an interview with Karen Tumulty of *Time* magazine in 2009, he stated: "We are not Europe. We are not Canada. We are America. This is not a single pay country."[16] When a hearing of health care reform options was to be considered before the Senate Finance Committee Round Table on Health Care in May 2009, eight activists from the single payer movement demanded a single payer voice at the 41-seat table. They entered the Senate chambers on May 5th for that purpose and made their request known. Senator Baucus' response—"We need more police." The eight were arrested, placed in handcuffs, charged with disorderly conduct/disrupting a congressional hearing, and taken off to jail. Though charges were later reduced, some community service was required of the "offenders." Some of the media picked up on the story. An avalanche of emails was received by MSNBC, and Dr. Margaret Flowers, a PNHP member from

TABLE 6.3

Public Opinion Concerning Possible Approaches to Health Care Reform

If you believe it is important to ensure access to affordable, high quality health care coverage and services for all Americans, which is most important to you? (SELECT ONE)

Meeting Site	Individual Tax Incentives	Expand Medicaid SCHIP, etc.	Rely on Free Market	Expand Medicare/ FEHBP	Expand Employer Tax Incentives	Expand Neighborhood Health clinics	Create a National Health Program	Individual Insurance Mandate	Increase State Program Flexibility
Albuquerque, NM	11.1%	2,5%	2.5%	3.7%	2.5%	4.9%	56.8%	6.2%	1.2%
Cincinnati, OH	7.8%	11.6%	6.0%	6.6%	3.9%	2.4%	39.7%	17.0%	0.6%
Fargo, ND	9.9%	7.7%	7.7%	5.5%	12.1%	3.3%	34.1%	9.9%	5.5%
Hartford, CT	0.0%	3.7%	0.0%	3.7%	3.7%	5.6%	74.1%	5.6%	0.0%
Las Vegas, NV	5.8%	7.2%	0.0%	8.7%	1.4%	2.9%	44.9%	20.3%	5.8%
Lexington, KY	6.3%	5.3%	3.2%	2.1%	2.1%	1.1%	54.7%	16.8%	0.0%
Little Rock, AR	11.9%	9.9%	1.0%	11.9%	5.0%	5.0%	25.7%	27.7%	1.0%
Los Angeles, CA	6.2%	6.2%	2.6%	7.2%	2.1%	6.7%	59.5%	3.6%	1.5%
San Antonio, TX	1.9%	4.9%	4.9%	5.8%	3.9%	1.0%	54.4%	19.4%	1.9%
Sioux Falls, SD	7.7%	11.5%	0.0%	15.4%	3.8%	0.0%	30.8%	23.1%	3.8%

Source: The Health Report to the American People. Report of the Citizens' Health Care Working Group. Appendix B, July 2006, available at http://www.govinfo.library.unt.edu/che/recommendations/appendix_html

Maryland, was featured as the leading story on *The Ed Show* shortly thereafter.[17]

The political debate over health care reform extended over a much longer period and with more dissention than the governing party, the Democrats, ever intended or anticipated. One target deadline after another was missed, giving more time and opportunity for opponents to mount opposition, slow down and even threaten reform altogether once the Democrats lost their filibuster proof majority in the Senate. As the debate wore on, often beyond the control of the parties themselves, the electorate and both major parties became more and more divided among themselves. In order to better understand these developments, it is useful to summarize them in three stages.

Before the August 2009 Congressional Recess

Figure 6.2 shows the results of a pre-recess poll by the Associated Press-GfK, with graphic evidence of increasing public disapproval of the Obama Administration's handling of health care over the first six months of his term.[18]

Republicans had a united front against most parts of the Democrats' health care proposals, ranging from opposition to a public option, mandates, costs of proposals to issues of fiscal responsibility, the role of government in health care, and burdens on the states by expanding Medicaid. The goal was to defeat ObamaCare, hand the new president a defeat on his number one domestic policy initiative, and position themselves for the 2010 elections. Their delicate balancing act, made more difficult by the lack of a counter proposal, was in achieving all that while not appearing to be obstructionist.

As the number two Republican in the Senate, Jon Kyl (R-AZ) stated his opposition to requiring all insurers to abandon policies denying coverage based on pre-existing conditions and to charge the same premiums regardless of health status, as well as requiring all Americans to purchase insurance. As he said:

"One of the concerns I have about the approach of the Democrats ... is an assumption that there has to be a national mandate on all insurers to do various things. Those are techniques that states can, and some have, used in the past with fairly disastrous consequences."[19]

FIGURE 6.2

Increased Opposition to Obama's Handling of Health Care

President Obama faces mounting resistance, particularly on Health Care

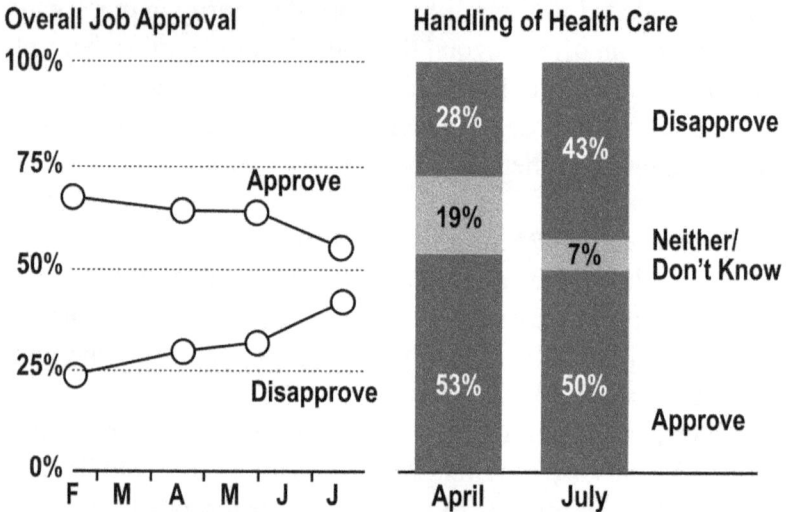

Source: Associated Press-Gfk telephone polls of at least 1,000 adults. Margin of error +/- 3.1 percentage points

Meanwhile, Democrats were experiencing increasing division among themselves over health care reform. In the House, the Blue Dogs, mostly conservative Democrats from the South, had become a pivotal swing power coalition with 52 members, about one-fifth of House Democratic members. Ironically, in their efforts to retake a majority in Congress in 2008, Democratic leaders had actively recruited moderate candidates in conservative districts. The Blue Dogs came back to bite the plans of more liberal and progressive Democrats, and threatened to vote against any health care bill that was too costly, too generous with subsidies, or disruptive to private insurers.[20]

After the August 2009 Congressional Recess

Concerned that his top domestic issue was losing momentum and that its opponents were gaining traction, President Obama gave a remarkable address to a Joint Session of Congress on September 9, 2009. As he sought to refocus the debate on the urgency of health care reform and build bipartisan support for bills taking shape in Congress, he had this to say:

> "I am not the first president to take up this cause, but I am determined to be the last. Our collective failure to meet this challenge—year after year, decade after decade—has led us to a breaking point."[21]

This address drew a national television audience of at least 32 million people. But despite its eloquence, it did little to change the nearly even split in public opinion and party differences over options of health care reform. In fact, a *USA Today*/Gallup poll taken a few days later showed that 60 percent of respondents believed bills in Congress would *not* accomplish the goals of reform, and many thought the bills would make the system's problems worse.[22] A *Wall Street Journal*/ NBC News poll in late September found that 45 percent of respondents approved of the way Obama and the Democrats were handling health care (vs. only 21 percent approval for Republicans in Congress).[23]

Even though clear majorities in these and other polls believed that the GOP's opposition to health care reform was politically motivated, rude and disrespectful, their attacks continued. The continual drumbeat was that Democratic health reforms would be bad for America. And their attacks were paying off. By late October, another *USA Today*/ Gallup poll found that only two in ten believed that the quality and costs of their own care would improve.[24]

Much as they tried to push back against the relentless GOP attacks, the Democrats had a difficult case to make. The President kept saying that any health care bill that would pass would not raise taxes or increase the deficit. Democrats claimed that the bill would be paid for by employers; individuals not purchasing insurance; cutbacks in Medicare spending; savings from such new initiatives as accountable care, prevention and wellness programs; and targeted taxes (the House favored a surtax on the wealthy, the Senate a tax on "Cadillac" insurance plans). But it soon became obvious to most people that a bill *would* require some pain for many taxpayers—the only questions were how much and for whom?

Then some new credible reports called into serious question claims by bill supporters that a bill would be deficit-neutral and would contain health care costs. The CBO found that middle-income Americans would end up paying higher insurance premiums, and that premiums would also be higher for those who gained coverage in a public plan through the Exchange. The CBO declined to count any cost savings for such pilot programs as prevention, wellness and accountable care organizations. And the CBO was quick to caution that its projections were so complex, with so many moving parts as changes to bills were added or deleted, that it could not assure their accuracy.[25]

But of course, many other contentious issues were in play at the same time, ranging from taxes on industry, levels of subsidies and for whom, coverage of abortion, and access to care among immigrants. United as the Republicans were against *any* health care bill, the Democrats were losing unity on many fronts, including cost of the program, impact on the deficit, use of federal funds for abortion, and how a public option, if there were to be one, would work. As Joshua Holland, editor and senior writer at *AlterNet* noted: "Within the Democrats' 'Big Tent', an incredibly significant game of chicken is being played."[26] That description held for various groups among Democrats in the House, such as who would vote for or against a watered-down public option or any amendments for abortion coverage, and how long each group would hold out.

After the November 2009 Elections

The November elections raised new questions about power relationships between the parties. The GOP won two governorships (New Jersey and Virginia) after a low turnout of Democratic voters and a majority of Independents voted for Republicans. All of a sudden the GOP was proclaiming its return to power. Representative Eric Cantor, the House Minority whip whose PAC was discussed in Chapter 2, declared: "[Voters are] looking for change... The Republican resurgence begins again tonight!" And a new Gallup poll reported that, in a generic Congressional matchup, Republicans moved ahead of the Democrats by 48 to 44 percent.[27]

The GOP was betting a lot on the health care bill. If it could kill the bill, it would win by showing how inept the Democratic majority was. If a bill passed that failed to contain costs and reform health care, they would also win by having actively opposed it. Since Democrats had a lot to lose either way, the stakes were raised another notch or two.

The Democrats were struggling to hold a fragmented coalition together. Forty-nine freshmen Democrats who won their House seats in red states carried by John McCain in the 2008 elections were more conservative than other Democrats on many issues, such as the role of government, abortion and gun control.[28] Some won their races by narrow margins, and would have to face re-election in 2010. Intense pressure was being put on all House Democrats to fall in line with their party. Thus, when it came down to the vote on H.R. 3962, all but the two co-sponsors of the single payer bill (H.R. 676) voted for the bill; only Reps. Dennis Kucinich (D-OH) and Eric Massa (D-NY) voted against it. Some factions were willing to kill the bill over their signature issue (e.g. the pro-life supporters through the Stupak amendment).

The Republicans were facing internal pressures as well. Underdogs were challenging the Republican Party's handpicked Senate candidates in several states. They were trying to take part in a wave of anti-establishment fervor. As one candidate, Rand Paul, a Senate candidate in Kentucky and son of the former presidential candidate Ron Paul, said: "There's a disconnect between the grassroots Republicans out here in the heartland and some of the leadership. I have yet to meet a Republican primary voter who would have voted for the bank bailout, and yet our leadership did."[29]

Then a mid-November report tossed even more fuel on the fire. The Center for Medicare and Medicaid Services (CMS) reported that the plan to cut some $500 billion from Medicare over ten years to help pay for the reform proposal would sharply reduce Medicare benefits for some seniors and compromise access to care for millions of others. This timely and well-done report was generated by the chief actuary of the Medicare program, and discredited the idea that Medicare cuts could be made to pay a large part of the costs of reform without jeopardizing access to physician and hospital care under the program.[30]

A November 17th ABC News/Gallup poll found that only 47 percent of respondents approved of President Obama's handling of the health care issue. Although 50 percent trusted the Democrats on health care (compared to 37 percent for Republicans), Independents were a larger group than either of the two major parties. From the beginning, Obama had taken a centrist and inconsistent approach toward health care reform. On the one hand, he acknowledged the need for major financing reform. He recognized the problems of the private health insurance industry, and had said:

> "If I were starting from scratch, I would build a system around single payer public financing."[31]

But after his election he never advocated a single payer approach, joining politicians assessing H.R. 676, the Conyers single payer bill already in the House, as politically infeasible. And when confronted by furious opposition from the insurance industry to his surrogate public option, seriously weakened by compromises in Congressional committees, he was quick to back down:

> "Whether we have [the public option] or we don't have it, is not the entirety of health care reform. This is just one sliver of it, one aspect of it … I don't want to put insurers out of business, just to keep them honest."[32]

After many months of bickering over the details of health care reform, public support for reform legislation drifted steadily downward. A mid-December *Wall Street Journal*/NBC News poll showed these striking results: 44 percent of respondents against passing a bill, only 41 percent for passage; 66 percent of liberal Democrats supportive, dropping from 81 percent three months previously. For the first time in his presidency, overall support for Obama fell below 50 percent.[33] At the same time, a tracking poll by the Kaiser Family Foundation found that only 35 percent of respondents said they would be personally better off after the passage of health care legislation, down from 42 percent a month earlier, and that one in four believed they would be *worse* off.[34]

And of course, as the debate raged on over a small public option and despite continued high public support for it, the political process killed that alternative in what finally was to come out of Congress. Dr. Margaret Flowers summed up the political dynamics in this insightful way:

> "In order to disarm the corporate interests, the health industries that had opposed previous reforms were included on the inside. In order to disarm the Right, bipartisanship was at the forefront. In order to disarm the supporters of a single payer plan, who are the majority, a campaign was developed around a promised

'compromise', the public option, and given tens of millions of dollars for organizing and advertising. The public option succeeded in splitting the single payer movement and confusing and distracting it with endless discussion about what type of public option would be effective."[35]

With this background of the forces seeking to exploit health care reform for their private interests, it is now time to see how all that played out over the 15 months culminating in the final bill passed by Congress and signed into law by President Obama in March 2010. Just how bad were the results of reform, anyway?

References

1. Flowers, M. After the reform: Aiming high for health justice. *Tikkun*, May/June 2010, p 15.
2. Steinmo, S, Watts, J. It's the institutions, stupid! Why comprehensive national health insurance always fails in America. *Journal of Health Politics, Policy and Law*, 20: 329, 1995.
3. Blendon, RJ, Benson, JM. Americans' views on health policy: A fifty-year historical perspective. *Health Affairs (Millwood)* 20 (2): 33, 2001.
4. Ibid # 3, p 35.
5. National Coalition on Healthcare. A report of a national survey. *Journal of Health Care Finance* 23: 12.
6. Hunt, AR. Public is split on how to pay for access. *Wall Street Journal*, June 25, 1998: A10.
7. Harris Interactive. Attitudes toward the United States health care system: Long-term trends—views of the public, employers, physicians, health plan managers are closer now than at any time in the past. Public Opinion Survey. *Harris Interactive*, 2 (17)
8. Press release. Commonwealth. New York. March 29, 2004.
9. PNHP. Recent public polls on single payer. The National Health Program Reader. Leadership Training Institute. October 24, 2008, pp 341-2.
10. Ibid # 9, p 342.
11. Horowitz, J. Winds of political change haven't shifted public's ideology balance. Pew Research Center Publications, November 28, 2008.
12. Zogby poll. American public remains divided over proposed healthcare reform. July 27, 2009.
13. E-mail communication between Kip Sullivan and Don McCanne, president of Physicians for a National Health Program, July 19, 2002.
14. The Health Report to the American People. Report of the Citizens' Health Care Working Group, Appendix B, July 2006, available at http://www.citizens health care.gov/recommendations/appendix_.pdf

15. Listen up! Asclepios. Your Weekly Medicare Consumer Advocacy Update. 6(32): August 10, 2006, p. 1.
16. Baucus, M. As quoted in interview with Karen Tumulty from *Time Magazine* in a Health Care Reform Newsmaker Series, March 3, 2009. Kaiser Family Foundation.
17. Robbins, K. Baucus 8 update: Single payer in the news. Healthcare-NOW! May 7, 2009. Available at http://www.healthcare-now.org/Baucus-8-update-single payer-in…
18. Zogby poll. American public remains divided over proposed healthcare reform. July 27, 2009.
19. Davis, T. Dem-GOP split on health care goes beyond public option. *ABC News*, August 19, 2009.
20. Bendavid, N. 'Blue Dog' Democrats hold health-care overhaul at bay. *Wall Street Journal*, July 27, 2009: A1.
21. Stolberg, SG, Zeleny, J. Says his health plan is necessary and will not add to the deficit. *New York Times*, September 10, 2009: A1.
22. Kaiser Health News, September 15, 2009.
23. Blow, CM. Obama's tortoise tactics. *New York Times*, October 23, 2009: A21.
24. Sussman, D. Skepticism about overhaul. *New York Times,* October 23, 2009: A22.
25. Adamy, J. House leaders unveil health bill. *Wall Street Journal*, October 30, 2009: A4.
26. Holland, J. Decent health care or an insurance industry bailout? *AlterNet*, November 3, 2009.
27. Blow, CM. The passion of the right. *New York Times*, November 14, 2009: A21.
28. Nagourney, A, Herszenhorn, DM. Trick for Democrats is juggling ideology and pragmatism. *New York Times,* November 10, 2009: A18.
29. Wallsten, P. Underdogs' Senate bids put pressure on GOP. *Wall Street Journal*, November 12, 2009: A8.
30. Montgomery, L. Report: Bill would reduce senior care. *Washington Post*, November 15, 2009.
31. PolitiFact. Truth-O-Meter. On a single payer health care system. Obama statements on single payer have changed a bit. July 1, 2009.
32. Williamson, E, Cole, A. Chances dim for a public plan. *Wall Street Journal*, August 17, 2009: A1.
33. Adamy, J. Support for health overhaul wanes. *Wall Street Journal*, December 17, 2009: A8.
34. Seelye, KQ. Ebbing public support. *New York Times*, December 19, 2009: A15.
35. Ibid # 1, p 14.

CHAPTER 7

Bailout Under a Blue Cross:
The Tortuous Path to a Gutted Bill in Congress

The debate over health care reform started well before the 2008 elections, and developed increasing intensity as the Obama administration came into office and set an initial urgent goal of delivering a health care reform bill in 2009. The debate ratcheted up to new highs as Congressional committees started to release their proposals and as each of many fine-print provisions came under attack. For those trying to track all these provisions in competing proposals, the task became daunting.

In previous chapters we have seen some of the powerful forces battling to preserve the status quo of our market-based system. Now it is time to see how the final legislation made its way through the sausage factory of Congress. There were many twists and turns as legislation was molded to be the least threatening to industry, and as the public interest was on many occasions neglected.

In his FY 2010 Budget overview, President Obama listed these principles as goals for health care reform:

- Reduce long-term growth of health care costs for businesses and government.
- Protect families from bankruptcy or debt because of health care costs.
- Guarantee choice of doctors and health plans.
- Invest in prevention and wellness.
- Assure affordable, quality health coverage for all Americans.
- Maintain coverage when you change or lose your job.
- End barriers to coverage for people with pre-existing medical conditions.

After setting forth these goals, the President left it up to Congress to fill in the details and come up with a bill.

THE FIRST THREE BILLS OUT OF THE HOPPER

The House took the initial lead in developing health care reform legislation, merging its three committees' bills into one, America's Affordable Health Choices Act of 2009 (H.R. 3200) by the end of July, before the August Congressional recess. Although the Democrats enjoyed a big majority in the House (256 to 178), votes in committee were close—no Republican support in any of the three committees and some Democrats voting against their party in each case, as shown in the following votes:

- House Education & Labor: 26 to 22 (3 Democrats opposed)
- House Ways & Means: 23 to 18 (3 Democrats opposed)
- House Energy & Commerce: 31 to 28 (5 Democrats opposed)

The Senate's Health, Education, Labor and Pensions Committee (HELP) released its Affordable Health Choices Act in July as well. The Senate Finance Committee (SFC) worked at a slower, more deliberate pace under the cloak of a quest for bipartisanship, hoping to persuade some of the three Republicans on its "Gang of Six" to vote for its bill. After Senator Baucus unveiled a blueprint of its plan in mid-September, all eyes shifted to the SFC as it dealt with some 564 amendments to the blueprint. Meanwhile, House leaders began to reassess how they might change their strategy in light of expected actions in the Senate.

The House bill (H.R. 3200) is a good starting point to understand the main elements, dimensions, and areas of controversy in reform legislation. In general, it was more liberal than proposals in the Senate, and probably represented the most that could be expected of any bill that might eventually be passed by Congress.

H.R. 3200 called for these basic elements:

- *Individual mandate*. All individuals would be required to have "acceptable health coverage" or pay a penalty; exemptions could be granted for dependents, religious objections and financial hardship.
- *Employer mandate*. Employers would be required to offer health insurance to their employees and contribute at least

72.5 percent of the premium cost for individual coverage and 65 percent of the cost of family coverage of the lowest cost plan that meets minimal benefits package requirements. Employers failing to comply would have to pay 8 percent of payroll into the Health Insurance Exchange Trust Fund. Subsequent Committee amendments provided for hardship exemptions for those employers that might face job losses as a result of this mandate, and eased requirements for small employers, exempting those with annual payrolls of less than $500,000 and reducing payments for those with payrolls between $500,000 and $750,000.

- *Health Insurance Exchange.* This would allow uninsured individuals and small employers to purchase qualified plans, both private and public. But those already covered by individual or employer-sponsored plans, as well as those on public programs such as Medicare, Medicaid, the VA, or TRICARE, would not have access to the Exchange.
- *Public option.* A new option to be offered through the Exchange that must meet the same requirements as private plans for benefit levels (basic, enhanced, premium and premium-plus), provider networks, cost-sharing and consumer protections.
- *Essential benefits package.* This package (yet to be defined and expected to produce intense controversy) would establish minimal requirements for plans offered through the Exchange. Then the multi-tiered coverage options would kick in as follows: the *basic* plan includes the minimal benefits package and covers 70 percent of the costs of the plan; the *enhanced* plan would reduce cost-sharing and covers 85 percent of benefit costs; a *premium* plan would also reduce cost-sharing and would cover 95 percent of benefit costs; and a *premium-plus* plan would provide additional benefits, such as dental health and vision care.
- *Individual subsidies.* Would provide "affordability premium credits" to eligible individuals and families with incomes up to 400 percent of the federal poverty level (FPL) ($88,000 in 2009 for a family of four). These credits would be based on the average cost of the three lowest cost basic health plans in the area, and would be set on a sliding scale basis relative

to income tiers (e.g. from 1.5 percent of income for those at 133 percent of FPL to 12 percent of income for those at 400 percent of FPL).

- *Employer subsidies.* Tax credits would be provided to employers with fewer than 25 employees and average wages of less than $40,000. The credits would vary in amount based on size of the firm and annual payrolls (e.g. employers with 10 or fewer employees and with average annual wages of $20,000 or less would receive credits for 50 percent of their premium costs; no tax credits would be provided for employees earning more than $80,000 a year).

- *Insurance reforms.* Guaranteed issue and renewability would be required, as well as elimination of pre-existing conditions as a basis for denial of coverage. Annual and lifetime caps would also be eliminated, and the Secretary of Health and Human Services would be empowered to limit health plans' medical loss ratios (MLRs) to a specified percentage. As we discuss elsewhere, this would mandate how much of each health care premium dollar would be spent on medical care.

- *Expansion of Medicaid.* Expanded Medicaid coverage would be extended to all individuals with incomes up to 133 percent of FPL. In addition, Medicaid payment rates would be increased to Medicare levels, and the federal government would pay the full costs of expansion through 2014.

- A new Center for Comparative Effectiveness Research would be created within the Agency for Healthcare Research and Quality to conduct, support and synthesize research on outcomes, effectiveness, and appropriateness of health care services and procedures.[1]

The bill proposed by the Senate's HELP Committee, the Affordable Health Choices Act, was similar in most respects to the House H.R. 3200 bill. These were the major differences:

- Various exemptions would be available to people unable to comply with the individual mandate, and penalties for non-compliance would be limited to $750 a year.

- Employers with more than 25 employees would be required to offer health coverage to their employees and contribute at least 60 percent of the premium cost or pay a penalty of $750 for each full-time employee or $375 for each part-time employee.
- Employer subsidies for small business were slightly more generous than provided by the House bill (e.g. employers with fewer than 50 employees and average wages of less than $50,000 would qualify for tax credits).
- Instead of a Health Insurance Exchange, state-based American Health Benefit Gateways would be created to serve the same purpose.
- Three benefit tiers would be offered by plans through the Gateways based on the percentage of allowed benefit costs covered by a plan. All three included the essential benefits package, but coverage of benefit costs would range from 76 percent for Tier 1 to 93 percent for Tier 3.
- Medicaid would be expanded to all individuals with incomes up to 150 percent of the federal poverty level (FPL).[2]

In mid-September, the Senate Finance Committee released its long-awaited bill after many months of heated debate behind closed doors. Chaired by Senator Max Baucus (D-MT), concerted efforts had been made to arrive at a bipartisan approach to a reform bill. These negotiations were carried out by the "Gang of Six," including three Republicans (Senators Michael Enzi /Wyoming, Charles Grassley / Iowa, and Olympia Snowe/Maine) and three Democrats (Senators Baucus, Kent Conrad/North Dakota, and Jeff Bingaman/New Mexico). After fractious bickering over many divisive issues, a bipartisan consensus was beyond reach.

The Baucus bill had some similarities to the Senate HELP and House bills, including an individual mandate starting in 2013, subsidies for individuals with incomes up to 300 percent of FPL, Health Insurance Exchanges where the uninsured and small business could shop for coverage, a ban on insurers from denying coverage because of pre-existing conditions, and Medicaid expansion beginning in 2014 for those with incomes below 133 percent of FPL. It did, however, have these important differences from competing proposals in the House and Senate:

- No employer mandate, though employers with more than 50 employees who are not providing coverage would be required to pay part of the cost of federal subsidies, up to $400 per worker.
- Individuals failing to purchase health insurance would pay penalties up to $3,800 a year.
- No public option; creation instead of nonprofit, member-run insurance cooperatives.
- Abortion could not be mandated as a covered benefit; use of tax credits to pay for abortion would be banned.
- A new tax would be imposed on insurers selling high-end Cadillac plans costing more than $8,000 for individuals and $21,000 for families.[3,4]

As expected, the Baucus bill was immediately controversial and open to attack from both the right and the left over a wide partisan divide. Within days after the Baucus plan was made public, 564 amendments were filed by legislators in both parties. On the right, examples included efforts to avoid an unfunded mandate for Medicaid expansion; reduction or elimination of fees imposed on insurance companies, clinical laboratories, and medical device manufacturers as a means of raising money to pay for subsidies; and prohibition of the use of federal money to pay for abortion.[5] On the left, supporters of the public option filed amendments to delete cooperatives as a way to compete with private insurers, while another amendment was intended to open up choice of new coverage to those already insured by other coverage.[6]

HOT-BUTTON ISSUES AS THE BATTLE HEATED UP

As Congress came back into session after its August recess with the three bills on the table as described above, the debate intensified with particular focus on the following hot-button issues:

- *Individual mandate.* This was fought by opponents as an assault on personal liberty, with some even questioning its constitutionality. The insurance industry pressed for a tight individual mandate with high enough penalties for non-compliance to discourage Americans from "going bare," which would reduce the potential value of a large risk pool as healthier people opted out.

- *Employer mandate.* Business was wary of the details of such a mandate. While small employers would gain from federal subsidies for their employees, large employers could end up paying more and losing some prerogatives they already had through the Employee Retirement Income and Security Act (ERISA).
- *Public option vs. co-ops.* Though most physicians and health professionals supported the public option, market stakeholders fought it like the plague.[7]
- *Subsidies.* Eligibility for subsidies was a hot topic. Liberals and progressives pushed harder to make insurance more affordable and for it to cover a higher proportion of health care costs, while conservatives pointed to an unending financial burden of a new entitlement program.
- *Cost of reform.* Could the reform package actually be deficit-neutral? The President's commitment to that goal was unpersuasive to most observers, and many saw projected savings in Medicare and Medicaid as "faith-based" and illusory.
- *Medicare cuts.* There was wide public support for reducing waste in the health care system. Eliminating overpayments averaging 14 percent higher to private Medicare Advantage plans should be a no-brainer, but the insurance industry fought such cuts, ironically backed by Republicans who were seeing themselves as defenders of seniors against the loss of private coverage to Medicare beneficiaries. The drug industry still feared negotiation of drug prices by the government, hoping that its pledge to offer a 50 percent rebate of drug costs in the doughnut hole would do the trick. Stakeholders demagogued the issue by fomenting fear among seniors that reform would bring cuts in their benefits.
- *Medicaid expansion.* States were increasingly worried about being given an unfunded mandate through health care reform, at a time when they were in desperate financial shape and unable to carry deficit budgets.
- *Insurance coverage.* Battles went on, mostly behind closed doors and receiving little coverage by the media, over such arcane but vital matters as the minimal benefit package to be required of insurers, how much of their costs they would be expected to pay, and whether the government would actually set MLR levels that

they must meet.
- *New taxes.* These were opposed by many groups, especially Republicans, Blue Dog Democrats and groups to be affected by such increases. Already those making over $500,000 a year had been identified for tax increases, as had insurers offering Cadillac plans.
- *Payment and reimbursement reform.* Physicians and many of their organizations pushed back against any threats to their income. The AMA warned that Medicare reimbursement rates would lead to a serious decline in the numbers of physicians accepting new Medicare patients. Interestingly, a just-released Government Accountability Office report found, contrary to this warning, that less than 3 percent of Medicare beneficiaries had major difficulties accessing physicians in 2007 and 2008, and that the willingness of physicians to serve Medicare patients and to accept Medicare reimbursement actually increased from 2000 to 2008.[8]
- *Use of cost-effectiveness research for coverage and reimbursement policy.* An army of stakeholders in the medical-industrial complex, together with their lobbyists (3,300 strong in the halls of Congress) continued to press their case that using cost-effectiveness in this way would limit innovation, slow medical progress, and damage the health of the public.

BUILDUP TO THE FLOOR VOTES

In The House

As the House moved toward finalizing its bill for a vote on the floor, the single most controversial issue was what to do about the public option. The original House bill (H.R. 3200) had called for a "robust" public option with payment rates tied to Medicare reimbursement rates for physicians and hospitals. Supporters held that such rates could put downward pressure on health care costs and force insurers to lower their premiums. Opponents included physicians and hospitals, who already felt under-reimbursed, as well as the insurance industry, which claimed it would be put out of business by competing against not-for-profit government coverage.

So politicians searched for other weaker, more politically palatable alternatives for the public option. In decreasing order of effectiveness (very limited already!), they came up with: the public option negotiating rates with providers and insurers; allowing states to opt out; and a delayed "trigger" to be used to activate a public option some years later only if cost containment goals were not achieved.

It was clear that there would be no Republican support for any kind of public option, and House Speaker Nancy Pelosi also knew that centrist and Blue Dog Democrats were likely to oppose the most robust option—premiums that amounted to Medicare rates plus 5 percent. When Senate Majority Leader Harry Reid announced that the Senate would move toward a public option in its merged bill, allowing states to opt out, Speaker Pelosi became more flexible on the public option. She bowed to centrist Democrats, gave up the Medicare plus 5 percent approach and put the public option forward based on negotiated rates. At the same time, she signaled that other options could be considered, even allowing states to opt out.[9]

Then, in order to break a logjam on the Energy and Commerce Committee, she cut a deal with New York Representative Anthony Weiner. In this deal, she backed down from a previous agreement granting liberals and progressives a floor vote on a single payer system.[10]

The New House Bill
H.R. 3962: The Affordable Health Care for America Act

With much fanfare, the new House bill was unveiled on October 29. As Speaker Pelosi said at the time: "We come before you to follow in the footsteps of those who gave our country Social Security and then Medicare."[11] That rhetorical overreach overlooked essential differences between the House bill, and Social Security and Medicare—those two programs were backed by the government *for all Americans* as part of a new social contract.

As expected, the new bill adjusted a number of details in an effort to broaden support among legislators with concerns over various provisions in the original bill. These are the main updates of the new bill (H.R. 3962) as compared with H.R. 3200:[12]

- *Individual mandate.* Starting in 2013, individuals would be required to purchase acceptable health insurance or pay a penalty of 2.5 percent of their income that is capped at the cost of the average cost of qualified coverage.

- *Employer mandate.* Starting in 2013, employers with annual payrolls more than $750,000 would be required to pay 8 percent of payroll if they fail to provide health coverage for their workers. Employers with annual payrolls between $500,000 and $750,000 would make smaller phased-in contributions. If coverage is unaffordable for low-wage workers, they could seek coverage through the Exchange, in which case employers would make their contributions to the Exchange.

- *Health Insurance Exchange.* A national Exchange would start in 2013, but states would have an option to start their own Exchanges if they meet federal standards. Initially, only the uninsured and small employers with 25 or fewer employees would have access to the Exchange. Employers with 50 or fewer employees would gain access to the Exchange in 2014, when the Exchange would also become available to those whose insurance premiums consume more than 12 percent of their family income. In 2015, the threshold for eligibility would increase to employers with 100 or fewer employees, and in later years, the Exchange could open up to larger employers.

- *Public option.* Starting in 2013, as described above. The CBO projected that the public option would cover only 6 million people by 2019, just 2 percent of Americans. The CBO also projected that the public option would cost more than private plans, since it would attract sicker individuals through adverse selection, could not set reimbursement rates for physicians and hospitals tied to Medicare rates, and would have to charge higher premiums. Moreover, it was projected that middle-income families might be required to spend 15 to 18 percent of their income on insurance premiums and co-payments.[13] The small weakened public option would not be able to have enough clout in the marketplace to be a competitive threat to private insurers.

- *Essential benefits package.* A Health Benefits Advisory Committee would be established in 2010 to provide recommendations to the Secretary of Health and Human Services on an essential benefits package. This committee would be chaired by the Surgeon General and include health care experts, health care providers and patients. A report to the Secretary of HHS would be expected in 2011 for adoption. Employers would not be required to meet the essential benefits package until 2018. Cost-sharing would vary across four tiers of coverage—*basic, standard, premium* and *premium plus*—from 70 percent for the basic plan to 95 percent for the premium plus plan. H.R. 3962 also called for creation of a new long-term care program (CLASS ACT), to supplement Medicaid and/or private long-term care insurance.

- *Individual subsidies.* These would be provided on a sliding-scale basis to individuals and families with incomes up to 400 percent of FPL.
- *Employer subsidies.* Small business tax credits would be provided for businesses with 10 or fewer employees and $20,000 or less in average wages. Credits would be phased out for employers with 25 or more employees or with average wages of $40,000 or more.
- *Insurance reforms.* Some reforms of current insurance industry practices would be introduced on a phased-in basis. In 2010, rescissions of coverage because of illness would be banned, as well as lifetime caps on coverage; young people could remain on their parents' coverage until their 27th birthday; individuals could keep their COBRA coverage until the Exchange is open in 2013; companies would be required to disclose rate increases for review; and MLRs would be set at a minimum of 85 percent (with a loophole probably crafted by insurance lobbyists "making sure that such a change doesn't further destabilize the current individual health insurance market"). In 2011, a three-year phase-down of Medicare Advantage overpayments would start, so that they would be at 100 percent fee-for-service reimbursement of traditional Medicare in 2014; at that time they would also be required to abide by a minimum MLR of 85 percent. In 2013, insurers would be prohibited from denying coverage because of pre-existing conditions, and would have limits on charging higher rates based on health status, gender or other factors, including a 2:1 maximum variation by age.
- *Expansion of Medicaid.* Eligibility for Medicaid would be expanded to 150 percent of FPL in 2013, with full federal funding for that expansion in 2013 and 2014; thereafter states would pay

9 percent of that cost. Some changes would be made to Medicaid before that, including elimination of cost-sharing for preventive services and increased reimbursement for primary care services in 2010.

- A Center for Comparative Effectiveness Research would be created at the Agency for Healthcare Research and Quality (AHRQ), but the bill "contained protections to ensure that research findings are not construed to mandate coverage, reimbursement or other policies to any public or private payer, and clarify that federal officers and employees will not interfere in the practice of medicine."

- The 1,990 page bill (almost 20-pounds) also included a number of other provisions, such as some improved benefits for early retirees; 12-month continuous eligibility for children in the States Children Insurance Program (SCHIP); revoking a decade-old anti-trust exemption for insurance companies; empowering the Secretary of HHS to negotiate prescription drug prices with manufacturers; requiring drug companies to give rebates for Medicare and Medicaid patients (amounting to $60 billion over ten years, in addition to the $80 billion in savings pledged earlier by the drug industry);[14] annual tax on manufacturers of medical devices of $20 billion;[15] contracts for studies by the Institute of Medicine on geographic variations of payment rates and health spending in the Medicare program; and funding for primary care workforce training programs in the 2015-2019 period.

The House had endeavored to keep the new bill under a target set by President Obama of $900 billion over ten years, and projected its *net* cost at $894 billion when first announced. That number was reached by separating out a bill for dealing with physician reimbursement under Medicare (the "doc fix"), estimated to cost some $247 billion over ten years. The CBO soon scored the new bill as costing $1.055 trillion in *gross* costs over ten years, while expressing reservations over the accuracy of its projections. About $425 billion would be spent over ten years to expand Medicaid and SCHIP, $605 billion for subsidies to low- and middle-income Americans to buy insurance on Exchanges, while $426 billion were estimated to accrue from cuts in Medicare and other federal health programs.[16]

Although President Obama welcomed the new bill as "an historic step forward," it immediately came under fire from all quarters. Republicans, of course, lambasted the bill as too expensive, not sustainable, adding too much bureaucracy and intrusion into health care, and even questioning the constitutionality of the individual mandate itself. They promptly moved to introduce their own, more limited bill including their pet favorites, such as state high-risk pools, malpractice liability reforms, and minimal regulation of insurers, but without individual and employer mandates, insurance reforms, expansion of Medicaid or new taxes.[17]

The Blue Dog coalition said that it needed more proof that long-term health care spending could be reined in. Karen Ignagni of AHIP stated: "We are not supportive of this bill in its current form. We think there is a missed opportunity on comprehensive cost containment." Hospitals, especially those in rural and affluent urban areas, feared cuts in reimbursement rates.[18] Employers said that the bill would saddle them with higher taxes, and physicians worried that they would be underpaid.[19]And business groups, including the National Federation of Independent Business and the U.S. Chamber of Commerce, began a multi-million-dollar TV ad campaign saying that the House bill would raise taxes and worsen the economy without containing health care expenses.[20]

House Speaker Pelosi planned to bring the bill to a floor vote within a week after it was announced. Although some stakeholders expressed support for the bill, including the AMA, the American Cancer Society, and AARP,[21] political turmoil was intense. Figure 7.1 shows how the debate played out for a number of groups in terms of how to pay for the bill. How to deal with abortion and the care of immigrants, both legal and illegal, remained highly controversial.

As time was running out to bring the bill to the floor before the Veterans Day holiday, and as the House leadership struggled to assure 218 votes for passage of the bill on the floor, Speaker Pelosi again decided *not* to allow a floor vote for the Wiener single payer amendment, which she had once promised. Although the Democratic majority in the House was then 258 to 177, it was clear that the vote on the floor would be very close. It appeared that at least eight Democrats would vote against the bill if they were given a chance to vote for the Wiener amendment. If she had allowed floor debate on single payer, the Speaker said she would also have had to permit debate of a Hyde

FIGURE 7.1

Who Pays?

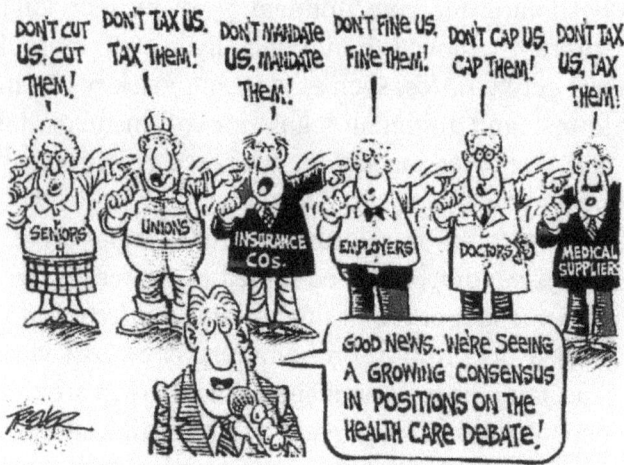

Source: Reprinted with permission of John Trever.

anti-abortion amendment, further delaying the process and perhaps threatening passage of H.R. 3962. Representative Weiner withdrew his amendment with this press release:

> "I have decided not to offer a single payer alternative to the health reform bill at this time. Given how fluid the negotiations are on the final push to get comprehensive health care reform that covers millions of Americans and contains costs through a public option, I became concerned that my amendment might undermine that important goal."[22]

As an example of the horse-trading that went on to gain to 218 votes, House leaders revised their bill to help certain doctor-owned specialty hospitals that serve large numbers of low-income Medicaid patients, in an effort to win the vote of Representative Harry Teague of New Mexico.[23]

The House bill was finally put to a floor vote on Saturday, November 7th. And as predicted, it was a cliffhanger all the way. It finally passed at 11:15 pm by a two vote margin of 220-215. Remarkably enough, the yeas included one lone Republican vote, that cast by Anh "Joseph" Cao (R-LA). Thirty-one of the 39 Democrats who voted against the bill were from districts that McCain won during the 2008 presidential election, with one-third of them freshmen Democrats from formerly Republican districts who considered themselves vulnerable in the 2010 elections.[24]

The bill would likely not have passed without Speaker Pelosi's concession the day before to allow a floor debate and vote on an anti-abortion amendment sponsored by Blue Dog Democrat Bart Stupak of Michigan. That amendment passed the next day by a vote of 240-194, assuring that no federal funds could be spent on abortion in the public option except in the case of rape, incest, or threat to the mother's life.

These two statements reflect the polarity of the final voting:

- Representative Cao (R-LA) said that he voted for the bill in order to "keep taxpayer dollars from funding abortion and to deliver access to affordable health care to the people of Louisiana."
- Representative Dennis Kucinich (D-OH), whose amendment that would have allowed individual states to create their own single payer systems was stripped from the House bill several days before at the request of the Obama Administration, had this to say: "Instead of working toward the elimination of for-profit insurance, H.R. 3962 will put the government in the role of accelerating the privatization of health care. In H.R. 3962, the government is requiring at least 21 million Americans to buy private health insurance from the very industry that causes costs to be so high, which will result in at least $70 billion in new annual revenue, much of which is coming from taxpayers. This inevitably will lead to even more costs, more subsidies, and higher profits for insurance companies—a bailout under a blue cross."[25]

Action by the House just before the Veterans Day holiday again shifted public attention back to the Senate, where the political pressures and stakes moved to even greater intensity.

In the Senate

It was clear from the start that the Senate would be a real challenge in getting a health care reform bill out of Congress and on to the President's desk. The Senate had been the graveyard for the Clinton Health Plan in 1994.

Although Senate Democrats had a potentially filibuster-proof majority of 60 (58 Democrats and 2 Independents), they included many moderates with serious concerns about the House bill. Senate Majority Leader Harry Reid (D-NV) would need 60 senators to vote for having a bill debated on the floor (which would likely involve weeks-long debate and political horse-trading). They could perhaps get the support of only one Republican—Senator Olympia Snowe (R-ME), but would have to meet the diverse needs of balking Democrats, including such moderates as Senator Mary Landrieu of Louisiana (where McCain won 59 percent of the vote in 2008), who was concerned about fiscal responsibility, help for teaching hospitals in her state, and care of foster children; Senator Evan Bayh of Indiana, who was very concerned about taxes on the medical device industry (an industry well established in his state); and Senator Blanche Lincoln (D-AR) (facing re-election in a red state where Obama lost by 20 points in 2008), with concerns about the cost of the House bill and the shortage of health providers in rural areas of her state.[26]

These are some of the amendments passed by the SFC over the weeks following the blueprint of the bill unveiled in mid-September:

- Reduce the maximum penalty for not complying with the individual mandate from $1,900 per family to $200 in 2014, phased up to $800 in 2017.
- Increase the threshold for payment of a tax by insurers for high-cost "Cadillac" plans from $21,000 to $26,000 for plans covering retirees and people in some high-risk occupations, such as fire fighters.
- Protect children from disruption of coverage under SCHIP.
- Protect Medicare patients with Medicare Advantage plans from loss of benefits.
- Prevent insurance companies from taking tax deductions for executive compensation above $500,000.
- Provide $1 billion in tax credits to biotech companies developing new therapies.[27]

Support of the reform effort by the insurance industry had been dropping off steadily as amendments loosened up the individual mandate. AHIP had commissioned a study by PricewaterhouseCoopers, releasing its results a few days before the SFC vote, which projected that a family health insurance policy costing $12,300 today would surge to an average of $25,900 by 2019 under this bill. AHIP followed up with ads warning seniors of loss of benefits with Medicare Advantage cutbacks (about $118 billion over ten years), while lobbying lawmakers that the industry's past cooperation was contingent on a tight individual mandate.[28]

The long-awaited vote in the Senate Finance Committee finally took place on October 14th, passing by a 14-9 vote, with one Republican supporter, Senator Olympia Snowe of Maine. The $829 billion package over ten years, as expected:

- liberalized the individual mandate by granting exemptions to people with religious objections and those unable to afford insurance;
- had no employer mandate (though employers with more than 50 employees would be required to help pay for government subsidies to their workers);
- would provide tax credits to small businesses with 25 or fewer employees;
- would substitute non-profit consumer-operated cooperatives for a public option;
- would expand Medicaid for individuals with incomes up to 133 percent of FPL;
- would phase out overpayments to Medicare Advantage plans; and
- would impose new fees on drug manufacturers and medical device makers ($23 billion and $40 billion over ten years, respectively).[29]

Merging the two Senate bills was not easy. The extent of disunity in the Senate next became obvious with the defeat of a Democratic initiative to increase payments to physicians by $247 billion over ten years (the "doc fix"). The test vote, needing 60 votes to proceed, went down 53-47 as twelve Democrats and one independent crossed party lines to vote with the Republicans. Proponents had hoped that its passage would increase physicians' support for their health care reform bill, while opponents saw this as fiscally irresponsible and a ploy to hide the cost of reform.[30]

Under growing pressure from the left and many moderates, Majority Leader Reid was struggling to hold together a weak coalition

of 58 Democrats and 2 Independents. In late October he indicated that
he was receptive to a public option that would be open to individuals
not covered by their employers but with a provision allowing states to
opt out. But that move just increased the pressure to meet the diverse
needs of conservative Democrats, and called into question whether the
Senate could act on health care reform before the end of the year, a
critical priority for the Obama Administration.

The fragility of the Democratic coalition in the Senate was
illustrated by the conflicting pressures on Senator Mary Landrieu of
Louisiana. On the one hand, 20 percent of her state's population was
uninsured and 25 percent were on Medicaid. She headed the Senate's
small business committee, and supported access by small employers to
an Exchange for their employees to get insurance. On the other hand,
she was being targeted by such groups as Conservatives for Patients'
Rights and Americans for Prosperity with ad campaigns and public
protests pushing her to "Kill the bill!"[31]

After narrow passage of the House bill (H.R. 3962) on November
7th, all eyes shifted to the Senate where lobbyists descended to target
their needs even more sharply. There was a considerable gap between
the House bill and the most conservative SFC bill, and political
observers were seeing a final Senate bill, *if* it were to pass, would likely
be close to the SFC bill.

The Merged Senate Bill

On November 18th, Senator Majority Leader Harry Reid released
the merged Senate bill, The Patient Protection and Affordable Care Act.
The 2,074 page bill was close to what was expected, including coming
in below the ten-year projected cost goal of $900 billion (at $848 billion), gained mostly by putting off many of its provisions until 2014,
raising new taxes, and cutting Medicare spending. The CBO said that
the bill would cut the deficit by $127 billion in the first ten years, with
further savings in the second decade. The bill called for a public option
allowing states to opt out; an increase in the Medicare payroll tax on
high-income people (individuals earning more than $200,000 a year,
$250,000 for couples); taxes on "Cadillac" plans costing more than
$8,500 a year for individuals and $23,000 for families); a requirement
that at least one insurance plan be available in every state covering
abortion (as well as one that does not); and a ban on illegal immigrants

purchasing insurance from a national exchange, even with their own money.[32]

The merged Senate bill faced a stormy course over the ensuing weeks as it was attacked by forces on both the right and the left. Republicans remained united in their efforts to further gut and kill the bill, while Democrats tried to hold their fragile coalition together. On November 21st, the Senate voted 60 to 39 along party lines to start debate on the bill after Thanksgiving, and the battle was joined with implications for the 2010 election campaigns.[33] These are some of the major amendments, compromises and developments over that tumultuous time:

- By a vote of 58-42, the Senate rejected a Republican amendment led by Senator John McCain that would have stripped some $400 billion in projected Medicare savings from the bill and sent it back to the Senate Finance Committee, effectively scuttling the bill. Disingenuously, Republicans postured as defenders of seniors, quite a switch from their many attempts over the years to limit or kill Medicare as an "out-of-control entitlement program." Shortly after that vote, as senators sought to reassure Medicare beneficiaries that their benefits would not be cut, they voted 100-0 for an amendment guaranteeing that a final bill would not cut their benefits.[34]
- A Republican amendment to eliminate the cuts to Medicare Advantage plans ($118 billion over ten years) was defeated 57-41.[35]
- As the controversy over federal funding of abortion heated up, an amendment offered by Senator Ben Nelson (D-NE) was defeated 54-45; the extent of division among the Democrats was exposed by seven Democrats voting with the Republicans.[36]
- Facing growing opposition to the bill on both sides of the aisle and increasing difficulty in getting 60 votes to move the bill forward, Senate Majority Leader Harry Reid announced a "broad agreement" compromise on December 9th whereby the public option would be eliminated and replaced by an expanded Medicare program allowing uninsured individuals between the ages of 55 and 64 to buy into Medicare.[37]
- The expanded Medicare option drew intense opposition from

organized medicine and hospitals, mostly due to fears of inadequate reimbursement. It soon became clear that there would not be 60 votes to move that forward, so it was removed from the bill in an effort to gain further support. Senator Joe Lieberman, "the Senator from Aetna," exercised the clout of his swing vote in killing that option, despite having campaigned for it in 2000 as a vice-presidential candidate. His assurances that his connections to the insurance industry had no influence over his vote strains credulity, since the Center for Responsive Politics reported that he received $684,344 in contributions from the insurance industry alone during the 2008 election cycle.[38]

- Two amendments close to the interests of the drug industry were defeated by narrow margins on December 15th as the pressure to reach enough consensus to allow a vote before Christmas became intense. The Senate voted 51-48 against a provision that would have allowed importation of cheaper prescription drugs from Canada and some other countries (60 votes were required for passage); a second provision was also defeated 56-43 that would have permitted imports only with a safety clearance by the FDA. Both votes met the goals of PhRMA, and curiously enough, the White House lobbied *for* these outcomes in order to maintain its "agreement" with PhRMA's $80 billion pledge made in the Spring, without which it feared losing the industry's support for reform.[39]

After compromising away some of the main provisions of the bill, such as the public option and the Medicare 55-64 expansion, Reid was still one vote short of the 60 needed to advance his bill—Senator Ben Nelson of Nebraska was still uncommitted, holding out for stronger anti-abortion language and concerned about the costs of Medicaid expansion.[40] As the revised bill (H.R. 3590) had been pulled incrementally to the right in an unsuccessful effort to appease its opponents, liberal and progressive Democrats were wavering in their support of the emasculated bill. With the loss of the Medicare buy-in and the public option, Howard Dean was calling for killing the bill in its tracks. In a courageous editorial, rare for the major media, MSNBC's Keith Olbermann called it as it was on December 16th:

"This is not health, this is not care, this is certainly not reform....

The 'men' of the current moment have lost to the 'mice' of history. They must now not make the defeat worse by passing a hollow shell of a bill just for the sake of a big-stage signing ceremony. This bill, slowly bled to death by the political equivalent of the leeches that were once thought state-of-the-art medicine, is now little more than a series of microscopically minor tweaks of a system which is the real-life, here-and-now version, or the malarkey of the Town Hallers. The American Insurance Cartel is the Death Panel, and this Senate bill does nothing to destroy it. Nor even to satiate it. ... Health care reform that benefits the industry at the cost of the people is intolerable and there are no moral constructs in which it can be supported."[41]

At a cost of about $100 million, Reid finally gained the vote of the last holdout, Senator Nelson, with further revision of the abortion language, exemption of Nebraska Blue Cross/Blue Shield and Mutual of Omaha's supplemental Medicare plan from taxes, and assurance that the federal government would pay 100 percent of the costs of Medicaid expansion in Nebraska *in perpetuity* (which was quickly dubbed the Cornhusker Kickback by envious senators). Getting the other holdouts off the fence was also expensive: Senator Mary Landrieu (D-LA) ($300 million in Medicaid subsidies for "certain states recovering from a medical disaster," such as Katrina); Senator Bill Nelson (D-FL) (grandfather clause that exempts Florida seniors currently on Medicare Advantage plans from losing those benefits, estimated at $3-5 billion); and Senator Bernie Sanders (I-VT), who negotiated $10 billion for community health centers, including $100 million in his own state.[42,43]

With 60 votes in hand, events moved quickly. Two procedural votes, won by the Democratic caucus at 60-40 and 60-39, culminated in the final vote on Christmas eve, by which the final Senate bill, with Reid's "manager's amendment," passed 60-39. Partisan wrangling began immediately, the Democrats touting their achievement as the most important legislation since Medicare and Social Security, and the Republicans decrying the bill as an "historic monstrosity" while vowing to continue the battle until the end.

Republicans had done all they could to delay action on the Senate bill, pulling out one procedural trick after another to prevent a floor vote before Christmas. When Senator Bernie Sanders of Vermont introduced his single payer, Medicare for All amendment No. 2837, they forced the entire 700-page amendment to be read aloud (which would have taken some ten hours). After almost three hours of its reading before a largely empty Senate, Sanders withdrew the amendment in exchange for 30 minutes of floor time. In his eloquent presentation that followed, he made clear that single payer national health insurance will *inevitably be required* in this country as the *only way* to assure universal access to comprehensive and cost-effective health care for all Americans, while at the same time reducing the waste and profiteering by private insurers and other corporate stakeholders in our enormous medical-industrial complex.[44]

FROM RECONCILIATION TO LAW OF THE LAND

The process then moved on to a conference committee to reconcile the differences between the two bills. At first, it was not clear how that was to be done, whether by a sizable joint committee or by negotiations between a few selected leaders in both chambers, most likely with active involvement by the White House. The second approach soon took over, with President Obama actively pushing for consensus. The reconciled bill would have to be passed by the chambers of Congress before going to the president for signature.

Because of the fragility of their 60 votes, the Senate leadership was wary of any significant changes from the Senate bill, but many liberals and progressives in the House felt betrayed by all the compromises made to secure passage by the Senate. Battle lines were still drawn over the public option, abortion, and ways to pay for the bill.

After a Congressional recess over the holidays, the battles over many divisive issues were rejoined and lobbyists went into overdrive for their final efforts to shape a bill to their liking. Negotiations were being carried out largely behind closed doors, generating Republican anger and public confusion about what might be in the final bill.

Meanwhile, stakeholders pressed their agendas—the AMA warned against the problems of bundled payments; AHIP kept fighting for a stronger individual mandate and more emphasis on containing health care costs, while continuing to oppose any regulation of premium rates; and the Catholic bishops, emboldened by their influence over wording of the Stupak amendment, even called for comatose patients with little hope of recovery to be given food, water and medicine.[45] But a wide partisan gap remained over many controversial issues between the two bills.

Then the Massachusetts bombshell changed the political landscape overnight. State Senator Scott Brown handed Democrat Martha Coakley a surprise defeat to fill the Senate seat of the recently deceased Senator Ted Kennedy after his 30-year career as a liberal leader of that body. Brown thereby became the 41st Republican vote in the Senate, terminating the filibuster-proof Democratic majority in the Senate and turning all bets for health care reform upside down. He had run a populist campaign, branding himself less a Republican and more an independent against the establishment, against too much intrusion of government, and resonating with unions and many middle class voters who had not seen the 2006 health care "reform" in their state reduce their health care costs. This turn-about event seemed to catch the Democratic party by surprise. Brown's 53-47 percent victory took place despite a last-minute visit by President Obama to the state in an unsuccessful attempt to breathe life into Coakley's campaign.

The Massachusetts election set off alarm bells throughout the Democratic establishment. Their ranks fell into confusion as they faced some daunting choices in trying to rescue the health care reform effort. Within days it became obvious that the House did not have the votes to pass even the Senate bill; the reconciliation process could only apply to budget matters; and a pared-down bill on "core elements" would likely be opposed by liberal Democrats. Democrats feared the repercussions of going away empty handed after more than a year of work on health care, but none of their options were promising. Obama scheduled a State of the Union address for January 27th, and signaled that he was open to a smaller bill.[46]

The tenor of the health care debate was completely changed after the Scott Brown victory in Massachusetts. Most believed that a major reform bill was dead in the water. Health insurance stocks surged after the news, Aetna rising by 4.2 percent and UnitedHealth by 4.1 percent; drug stocks also rebounded, Merck making the biggest advance among the 30 stocks that make up the Dow Jones industrials.[47]

The State of the Union address on January 27th did not alter the political landscape. The major focus was on jobs; health care was not even mentioned until more than a half hour had elapsed, and the President offered no clear way forward on the impasse over health care reform. His assertion that he would "keep fighting for health care reform" came across as unpersuasive rhetoric, especially when he put out this challenge to critics of the health care bills: "If anyone from either party has a better approach that will bring down premiums, bring down the deficit, cover the uninsured, strengthen Medicare for seniors and stop insurance company abuses, let me know."[48]

The next morning, Dr. Margaret Flowers, member of the Baucus Eight whom we met in the last chapter, sent an open letter to President Obama detailing how a single payer system, Medicare for All could do all those things. She requested that the President meet with representatives of the Leadership Conference for Guaranteed Health Care, a coalition of nurses, physicians, and health care advocates. As expected, this request was rebuffed by the White House.[49]

As January drew to a close, the prevailing view was that health care was on life support, and that a comprehensive bill could not be passed in the election year. Reconciliation appeared dead as three centrist Senate Democrats announced they would oppose that approach to get around the need for 60 votes. There were still calls to break up the bills and try to pass portions as "core elements," but which elements should be picked?

Meanwhile, as hopes dimmed for health care reform, the blame game took on new energy. Many members of Congress blamed the President for lack of leadership and clear direction, Republicans noted that a majority of the electorate was against the reform bills, Independents had voted against reform in Massachusetts, Democrats were too divided to see their way forward, though still reluctant to declare reform dead.

But more was to come. In a pullback from the brink of defeat, Democrats and the Obama Administration were faced with some major decisions—whether to press on with a comprehensive reform bill or break it up into smaller pieces, and how to deal with the loss of a 60-vote Senate majority after the win of Republican Scott Brown in Massachusetts. Confronted by these new realities, re-energized Democrats rapidly developed some new strategies for the end game in Congress.

Obama took a more active role in an attempt to unify the Democratic majority for health care reform, based mostly on the most conservative version—the Senate bill. He set a new hard deadline for the passage of health care reform legislation by the end of March, to be preceded by an all-day bipartisan Health Care Summit of leaders of both parties and the Administration in Washington, D.C. on February 26th.

In advance of the Summit, the President released his proposal, a $950 billion proposal over ten years, very similar to the Senate bill, but with the differences shown in Table 7.1.[50]

But, as widely predicted, the summit was a failure in terms of policy substance. Both sides used it as a forum to rehash their differences, there were no concessions from either party, and many statements were made that did not pass fact-checks. A post-Summit assessment was that the all-day televised session did not bridge partisan divisions, but even made them farther apart.[51]

In an attempt to avoid a Senate filibuster, Democratic leaders decided on a strategy to include final revisions in a budget reconciliation bill, which could be adopted by a simple majority in both the House and Senate. First, the House had to pass the Senate bill, which had been passed on Christmas eve, despite their reservations, but with enough assurances that the Senate would then pass a companion bill to fix their concerns about the Senate bill. Recent changes in the House membership had brought the magic number to 216 for a House majority of the then 431 House members.

The end game in Congress then entered its climactic finale. Both opponents and supporters of health reform legislation made their final push to influence pivotal swing votes. Leading the opposition were the U.S. Chamber of Commerce and such groups as Americans for Prosperity; supporters of reform included the drug industry, labor unions and other groups.[52]

The budget reconciliation bill would reduce the Senate's tax on high-cost insurance plans, increase subsidies to help lower-income people buy health insurance, and increase the Medicare payroll tax on wages as well as extend it to unearned income for affluent taxpayers. The CBO gave the measure further momentum by releasing an updated report that the revised Senate-passed bill would spend $940 billion to gain coverage for 32 million uninsured people over the next ten years, while reducing the deficit by $138 billion.[53]

As the political drama over health care reached its zenith, President Obama issued a last-minute exhortatory effort to get a bill out of Congress. In his *"This is it"* speech on March 3rd, the President had

TABLE 7.1

Obama Plan: How the President's Plan Stacked Up to the Senate Bill

	Tax on high-value insurance plans	Mandate on individuals	Employer mandate	Regulating premiums	Fees on drug makers
Obama	Insurance plans valued at more than $27,500 for a family would face a 40% tax starting in 2018.	People who refuse to carry health insurance pay up to 25% of income as penalty. Exemption for lower-income people.	Employers with 50 or more workers pay fine of up to $2000 per worker if they fail to offer coverage and workers get government subsidies.	New federal body would have power to block insurers from raising rates.	$33 billion over 10 years
Senate	Started tax five years earlier and set threshold at $23000	Similar, but maximum penalty was 2.0% of income.	Similar, but fine was capped at $750 per worker.	No such body created.	$23 billion over 10 years
Comment	Tax is unpopular among unions and liberal Democrats. The White House announced an agreement delaying the tax only for unions, but the proposal released applies to all workers.	Critics say the mandate was unconstitutional; supporters say it is needed to get healthy customers into the insurance pool.	Proposal was opposed by business groups.	Obama responds to recent sharp rate increases by WellPoint and others.	Chief drug lobbyist who negotiated the lower fees announced his resignation

Source: Adamy, J., Meckler, L. Obama renews health push. *Wall Street Journal*, February 23, 2010: A1.

this to say:

> "On one end of the spectrum, there are some who have suggested scrapping our system of private insurance and replacing it with government-run health care. Though many other countries have such a system, in America it would be neither practical nor realistic... I don't believe we should give government bureaucrats or insurance company bureaucrats more control over health care in America."[54]

As Matthew Rothschild, editor of *The Progressive* points out:

> "By damning 'government bureaucrats,' Obama played right into the hands of the anti-government crowd and made any durable expansion of health care coverage all the more difficult. He also cast aspersions on every single federal employee in the Medicare and Medicaid and VA and Indian health programs. Single payer advocates like you and me were props for him all along."[55]

News cycles were filled with attention to the unfolding health care drama, and it was uncertain how it would end. Obama delayed a trip to Indonesia and Australia in order to be available to bring last-minute pressure on legislators on the fence.[56] It was widely expected to be a close call, and it was. Compared to the long journey of potential bills over some 15 months, the last days were rapid and decisive, as these votes took place to pass the Health Care and Education Affordability Reconciliation Act of 2010 (H.R. 4872) by narrow margins:

- In the House, on March 21st—by 219-212
- In the Senate, on March 24th—by 56-43, with three Democrats voting with the Republicans (Senators Ben Nelson of Nebraska, and Blanche Lincoln and Mark Pryor of Arkansas)
- In the House again, on March 25th—by 220-207

Health care "reform" 2010 became the law of the land, hailed by its supporters as an historic breakthrough of the magnitude of Social Security, Medicare and the civil rights movement. But just what did we get in terms of value? That is the subject of the next chapter.

References

1.   Focus on Health Reform. Side-by-side comparison of major health care reform proposals. Kaiser Family Foundation. Accessed August 5, 2009 at www.kff.org.
2.   Ibid # 1.
3.   Hulse, C. For Senate Democrats, 60 is the magic number. *New York Times*, September 17, 2009: A 20.
4.   Hitt, G, Adamy, J, Weisman, J. Senate bill sets lines for health showdown. *Wall Street Journal*, September 17, 2009: A 1.
5.   Pear, R, Herszenhorn, DM. New objections to Baucus health care proposal. *New York Times*, September 15, 2009: A 23.
6.   Herszenhorn, DM. Prescriptions. Democrat vs. Democrat. *New York Times*, September 23, 2009: A 20.
7.   .Building a National Insurance Exchange: Lessons from California. Issue Brief, California HealthCare Foundation, July 2009.
8.   GAO. Medicare physician services. Utilization trends indicate sustained beneficiary access with high and growing levels of service in some areas of the nation. August 2009.
9.   Pear, R, Herszenhorn, DM. Pelosi intensifies pressure on House Democrats for government insurance plan. *New York Times*, October 24, 2009: A 10.
10.   O'Connor, P, Frates, C. Nancy Pelosi starts clock on House health bill. *Politico*, October 29, 2009.
11.   Adamy, J. House leaders unveil health bill. *Wall Street Journal*, October 30, 2009: A4.
12.   Summary prepared by House Committees on Ways & Means, Energy & Commerce, and Education & Labor, October 29, 2009.
13.   Medical News Today and *New York Times*. CBO: House health bill would lower some middle class premiums, raise costs for others. November 4, 2009.
14.   Mundy, A. Drug makers face tougher measures. *Wall Street Journal*, October 30, 2009: A4.
15.   Ibid # 14.
16.   Ibid # 11.
17.   Pear, R, Herszenhorn, DM. G.O.P. counters with a health plan of its own. *New York Times*, November 4, 2009: A18.
18.   Hartocollis, A. Hospitals cite worries on fees in health bill. *New York Times*, November 3, 2009: A1.
19.   Ibid # 11.
20.   Kaiser Health News. November 3, 2009.
21.   Bendavid, N, Adamy, J. Health bill garners endorsements. *Wall Street Journal*, November 6, 2009: A8)
22.   Wiener, A. Press release. Representative Wiener withdraws single payer amendment from current health care debate.
23.   Hulse, C, Herszenhorn, DM. House Democrats seek allies for health care vote. *New York Times*, November 6, 2009: A15.
24.   Leopold, J. House passes sweeping health care reform legislation. *Truthout*, November 8, 2009.

25. Ibid # 24.
26. Bendavid, N. Democrats pose health bill hurdle. *Wall Street Journal,* November 6, 2009: A1.
27. Pear, R, Herszenhorn, DM. Finance panel wraps up its work on health care bill.
    New York Times, October 3, 2009: A16.
28. Johnson, A. Insurers stand against committee's plan. *Wall Street Journal,* October
14. 2009: A5.
29. Pear, R, Herszenhorn, DM. A Senate health bill gains with one Republican vote. *New York Times*, October 14, 2009: A1.
30. Pear, R, Herszenhorn, DM. Democrats lose big test vote on health legislation. *New York Times*, October 22, 2009: A21.
31. Bendavid, N. Democrats pose health bill hurdle. *Wall Street Journal,* November 6, 2009: A1.
32. Pear, R, Herszenhorn, DM. Senate leaders unveil measure on health care. *New York Times*, November 19, 2009: A1)
33. Silva, M. Reaction to Senate healthcare vote offers a preview of 2010 campaigns.*Los Angeles Times*, November 23, 2009.
34. Pear, R, Herszenhorn, DM. Senate backs preventive care for women. *New York Times*, December 4, 2009: A20.
35. Pear, R, Herszenhorn, DM. Efforts to strip health care provisions fall short. *New York Times*, December 5, 2009: A13.
36. Hook, J, Levey, NN. Senate Democrats reach healthcare deal on 'public option'.*Los Angeles Times*, December 9, 2009.
37. Ibid #36.
38. Bendavid, N, Yoest, P. Lieberman's ties to ex-party frayed by his use of swing vote. *New York Times,* December 16, 2009: A7)
39. Mundy, A. Drug-import bill rejected by Senate. *Wall Street Journal*, December 16, 2009: A7.
40. Hitt, G. Reid fights for 60th vote on health bill. *Wall Street Journal*, December 17, 2009: A4.
41. Olbermann, K. Special comment: Not health, not care, not reform. MSNBC on December 16, 2009, as well as on Daily KOS blog on that date.
42. Bendavid, N, Adamy, J, Johnson, A. Republicans take aim at deal-making. *Wall Street Journal*, December 22, 2009: A5.
43. Editorial. The price of 'history'. *Wall Street Journal*, December 23, 2009: A20.
44. Smith, D. Sanders says single payer day will come as he withdraws amendment.Healthcare-NOW! December 17, 2009. Accessed at http://www. healthcare-now.org/sanders-says-single payer-day-wil...
45. Egelko, B. New Catholic mandate on comatose patients. *San Francisco Chronicle*, January 4, 2010.
46. Stolberg, SG, Herszenhorn, DM. Obama weighs a paring of goals for a health bill. *New York Times*, January 21, 2010: A1.

47. Paradis, T. Mass. vote pulls health stocks up. Associated Press, January 20, 2010.
48. Obama, B. State of the Union Address, Washington, D.C. January 27, 2010.
49. Flowers, M. An open letter to President Obama on health care reform. January 28, 2010.
50. Adamy, J, Meckler, L. Obama renews health push. *Wall Street Journal*, February 23, 2010: A1.
51. Stolberg, SG, Pear, R. Health meeting fails to bridge partisan rift. *New York Times*, February 26, 2010: A1.
52. Zeleny, J. Millions being spent to sway Democrats on health care bill. *New York Times*, March 13, 2010: A1.
53. Hitt, G, Adamy, J. Health showdown is set. *Wall Street Journal,* March 19, 2010: A1.
54. Rothschild, M. The Molly Ivans story. *The Progressive* 74 (4): 4. April 2010.
55. Ibid # 54.
56. Hitt, G, Adamy, J. Health-care end game begins. *Wall Street Journal*, March 13,2010: A4.

PART II

Where is Health Care "Reform" 2010 Taking Us?

CHAPTER 8

Health Care "Reform" 2010:
Better Than Nothing?

"Our health care system has not been cured or even stabilized. For now, we will continue to practice under a financing system that obstructs good patient care and squanders vast resources on profit and bureaucracy. Passage of the health reform law was a major political event. But for most doctors and patients it's no big deal."
                    —David Himmelstein, M.D. and Steffie Woolhandler, M.D.,
                    co-founders of Physicians for a National Health Program[1]

Now that it has passed, will the health care law meet our health care needs or not? And how does it stack up against a simpler proposal, Medicare for All? This chapter will answer both questions by (1) showing how the new health care legislation, despite a number of salutary provisions, will fail to effectively address the main priorities of reform; and (2) comparing this version of health care "reform" with a not-for-profit publicly financed system coupled with a private delivery system, an improved Medicare for All.

WILL THIS MULTI-PAYER "REFORM" BILL WORK?

In order to assess its long-term effectiveness as a reform bill, we need to return to the three major goals of reform: (1) to contain rapidly escalating costs of health care and insurance, making them more affordable; (2) to expand access to the entire population; and (3) to improve the quality of care. As we have already seen, addressing each of these goals requires addressing many interrelated factors. For example, you cannot control costs without system accountability, limiting wasteful bureaucracy, and reining in unnecessary and inappropriate services. And you can't improve quality of care unless all Americans have affordable access to necessary care, with insurance coverage for most of those costs.

The Good News

On the plus side, the new health care reform legislation brought forward this impressive list of steps:

- extending health insurance to 32 million more people by 2019;
- subsidies to help lower-income people to afford health insurance;
- allowance for parents to keep their children on their policies until age 26;
- expansion of Medicaid to cover 16 million more lower-income Americans;
- $11 billion new funding for community health centers that could enable them to nearly double their current patient volume;
- coverage without cost-sharing of preventive services recommended by the U.S. Preventive Services Task Force, together with an annual wellness visit and a personalized prevention plan;
- phasing out by 2020 the "doughnut hole" coverage gap for the Medicare prescription drug benefit;
- creation of a new voluntary national insurance program for long-term services: Community Living Assistance Services and Supports (CLASS) program;
- creation of a non-profit Patient-Centered Outcomes Research Institute charged with examining the relative outcomes, clinical effectiveness and appropriateness of different medical treatments;
- initiating some limited reforms of the insurance industry, including prohibition of pre-existing condition exclusions and banning of annual and lifetime limits; and
- providing a 10 percent bonus for primary care physicians, together with some provisions to expand the primary care workforce.

The Bad News: More Failed Health Care Legislation

Many people thought the above steps forward made this law worth it, usually followed by such statements as "the perfect is the enemy of the good," more rigorous reform "just wasn't politically feasible," or "this is a good start that we can improve on later". But this list of incremental improvements would not have been necessary had more fundamental system reform been undertaken, particularly by replacing the wasteful profit-driven private insurance industry with a not-for-profit public financing system, an improved Medicare for All. Moreover, most of the above incremental steps could have been enacted separately without attaching them to a massive "overhaul" bill that was served up to us by market-based corporate stakeholders, their allies and willing politicians.

Admittedly, our health care system is immensely complicated, and there are good reasons why serious reform attempts have failed on many occasions in the past. Despite the present hyperbole by its supporters, this latest effort will end up as just another failed reform effort littering the landscape of the last century. Cutting through the thicket of complexity, these are the most important ways in which the new health care "reform" law will fail the basic goals of reform. Considering these points, you can then decide for yourself whether you think this is a good law or not.

1. *Surging costs of health care and insurance will not be contained.*

Here are some of the ways by which health care costs will continue to increase at several times the rates of cost-of-living and median wages:

- No price controls; Wall Street has already factored in rapid expansions of markets for drugs, medical devices and other services in a system of expanded access—health care stocks rose more than 28 percent in less than three months after Congress released the first of its health care bills on October 30, 2009.[2]
- No bulk purchasing, such as is done so well by the Veterans Administration; the new law has banned a role of the government in negotiating prices of prescription drugs and prohibited importation of drugs from Canada and other countries.
- Lack of controls over perverse incentives that drive increased volume of unnecessary and inappropriate services. These are encouraged by retention of fee-for-service (FFS) reimbursement and weak coverage policies whereby many services are not subject to rigorous evidence-based criteria for efficacy and cost-

effectiveness. The long-delayed experiments with accountable care organizations (ACOs) and bundled payments are much too little and too late to be effective. While integrated systems like Kaiser Permanente, Group Health Care Cooperative and the Mayo Clinic are good cost-control models, they rely on *salaried* physicians without incentives to increase volume. The new law has grandfathered-in specialty hospitals, typically physician-owned facilities allowing physicians to "triple-dip," increasing their incomes as providers, owners and investors.

- The "doc fix" was not included in the final bill, partly as a ploy to keep the apparent 10-year cost of the bill under $1 trillion. But we can be sure that medical organizations will strongly resist any cuts in their present reimbursement, already excessively high for many specialized procedures. This was recently demonstrated by plastic surgeons pushing back and the AMA successfully preventing a 5 percent tax on elective plastic surgery from becoming part of the Senate bill (soon dubbed the "Botax" after the anti-wrinkle product Botox).[3,4]

- The bill will not alter the dominant business model of health care, whereby health care is a commodity, many facilities and services are for-profit and investor-owned, and emphasis on financial bottom lines and returns to shareholders often trump the public interest.

- While coverage of preventive services is a welcome addition in the new law, increased emphasis on prevention won't save money, but will *increase* health care costs due to diagnostic and treatment services engendered.[5]

- Many other parts of the medical-industrial complex are gearing up for increased profits from expanded subsidized coverage. We can expect each to add more to the cost of care than is presently anticipated. A good example is in the area of health information technology (HIT). Although some proponents tell us that HIT can save money through new efficiencies, the opposite is far more likely.[6]

- Private insurers can't contain health care costs, even in areas where they have dominant market power. In fact, the opposite is well documented. In November 2009, the Congressional Research Service released a report, *The Market Structure of the*

Health Insurance Industry, which concluded that: "The exercise of market power by firms in concentrated markets generally leads to higher prices and reduced output—high premiums and limited access to health insurance—combined with high profits."[7]

- The reform bill has no effective way of reining in the adoption of marginal or ineffective technologies. One current example is widespread adoption of 64-slice CT cardiac scanners with little evidence of their clinical value, possible increased cancer risks from radiation exposure, and with strong evidence that many hospitals adopt this procedure to increase their revenue streams.[8] The new Patient-Centered Outcomes Research Institute will not have the power to mandate or even endorse coverage or reimbursement rules for any particular treatment.[9]

- In our current market-based system, there is little incentive for physicians and hospitals to cut down on inappropriate or unnecessary services that raise their incomes; the new law doesn't change that.[10]

- The bill will not restrain premium increases. Because the individual mandate was attenuated, with lowered penalties for those choosing to remain uninsured, insurers will not gain the expanded markets that they were hoping for. They will still have many ways to maintain their profits, including continued escalation of premiums for policies with less coverage. Premiums for the much-touted Federal Employees Health Benefits Plan (FEHBP) increased by 8.8 percent in 2010.[11] The health insurance industry is already dependent on government subsidies for its survival. The stark projection of how quickly premiums are expected to become unaffordable for most of the population is shown by Figure 8.1.[12]

- In the midst of a prolonged recession, and a weak job market with blunted earning potential, $476 billion in new public subsidies over ten years will stress government coffers likely to the point of being unsustainable.[13]

- Smoke and mirrors in budget projections have made future health care costs look smaller than they will be. For starters, most of the benefits under the Senate bill will not come on line until

FIGURE 8.1

Annual Health Insurance Premiums and Household Income, 1996 to 2025

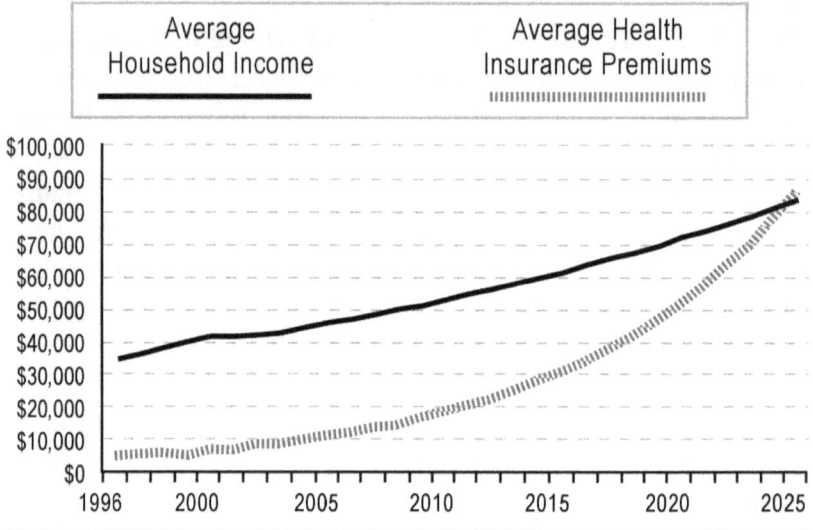

Source: Reprinted with permission from: Graham Center One-Pager. Who will have health insurance in 2025? *Am Fam Physician* 72(10):2005.

2014 (another ploy to get a "good" CBO score and keep the 10-year cost within an approvable range for legislators). About one-half of the program will be financed by Medicare cuts and other "savings" in the program. But these have still not been made clear, and the CBO has found that they were double-counted. As Richard Foster, the chief Medicare actuary said: "The same money cannot be simultaneously used to cover the uninsured and to extend the Medicare trust fund, despite the appearance of this result from the respective accounting conventions."[14] And as the well-known business columnist Robert Samuelson reminds us: "The word 'savings' is misused when it implies actual reductions—when it just signifies smaller future increases."[15]

• Although the final bill has authorized an independent commission to recommend some limitations in Medicare reimbursement rates for some services, these will be difficult to enforce and will apply only to about one-sixth of the overall health care system.

National health expenditures, now more than $2.5 trillion a year ($8,289 per capita), already consume 17.3 percent of the GDP.[16] In view of the above factors, costs of health care will continue upward unabated and will likely sink the boats of an increasing part of our population, as illustrated by Figure 8.2.[17]

The CBO projects that the $1.1 trillion health care plan will be paid for by spending cuts (49 percent) and new taxes and fees (51 percent). Of that total, $965 billion will be spent on the plan, including 45

FIGURE 8.2

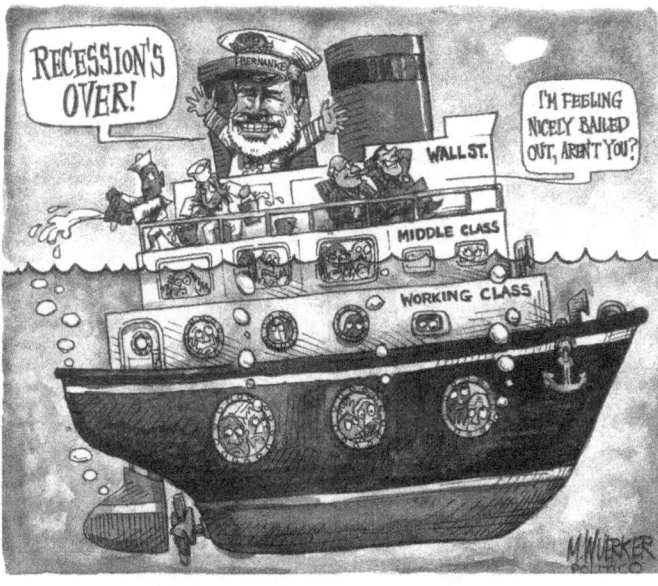

Sinking Ship of the Middle Class

Source: Reprinted with permission of Matt Wuerker.

percent for Medicaid and SCHIP and 47 percent on premium and cost-sharing subsidies. The remaining $135 billion will be used to decrease the deficit.[18] But as the CBO readily acknowledges, these projections are fraught with uncertainty. They may end up costing much more than estimated today. For example, any future Medicare cuts will be hard-fought by many constituencies, so that source of funding for the reform law may fall considerably short of projections.

2. *Uncontrolled costs of health care and insurance will make them unaffordable for a large and growing part of the population.*

We have been told from the beginning that health care reform will control costs and make health care more affordable for American families. In his election campaign, Obama promised that costs would go down by about $2,500 a year for the average family. And the reform bill allocates $476 billion for subsidies to help make these costs affordable. But is that real?

Won't all these subsidies help? Examined more closely, the answer turns out to be not as much as we might think. For starters, subsidies will not be available to anyone already covered by employer-sponsored insurance, those eligible for Medicaid (less than 133 percent of FPL) and those with incomes more than 400 percent of FPL. And subsidies can only be obtained by purchasing coverage on their own on an Exchange, to be set up in 2014. A rough idea of how these subsidies will likely sort out is shown in Table 8.1 (based on the earlier Senate bill). But these estimates are overly optimistic since they are based on 2009 premium levels, certain to be much higher by 2014.[19]

If we take as an example a typical family of four in 2016, with a 40-year old head of household with annual family income of $60,000 (250 percent of FPL), we find that subsidies will help considerably with payment of premiums, but will provide little protection against high annual out-of-pocket costs. Most experts consider health care costs above 10 percent of annual family income to be a financial hardship and difficult for most families to afford.[20] So in this case, according to projections by MIT's Jonathan Gruber and CBO cost estimates, this family would be at risk for up to 20 percent of family income (Table 8.2).[21,22]

Here are several ways in which the reform bill will *not* make health care more affordable:

- Insurers can increase premiums based on age (by a 3 to 1 ratio), geographic area, tobacco use (by a 1.5 to 1 ratio), and by the number of family members.
- Increased cost-sharing requirements for those covered by employer-sponsored insurance; as employers find themselves saddled with higher health care costs, their typical response will

TABLE 8.1

Payments and Subsidies Under Senate Bill

What the Person/Family Pays by Age and Income

	20	30	40	50	60
150%	$1,505	$1,505	$1,505	$1,505	$1,505
175%	$2,093	$2,093	$2,093	$2,093	$2,093
200%	$2,778	$2,778	$2,778	$2,778	$2,778
225%	$3,560	$3,560	$3,560	$3,560	$3,560
250%	$4,438	$4,438	$4,438	$4,438	$4,438
275%	$5,412	$5,412	$5,412	$5,412	$5,412
300%	$6,483	$6,483	$6,483	$6,483	$6,483
325%	$7,023	$7,023	$7,023	$7,023	$7,023
350%	$7,108	$7,563	$7,563	$7,563	$7,563
375%	$7,108	$7,862	$8,103	$8,103	$8,103
400%	$7,108	$7,862	$8,644	$8,644	$8,644

Subsidy Amounts

	20	30	40	50	60
150%	$5,604	$6,357	$7,930	$11,607	$17,195
175%	$5,015	$5,769	$7,341	$11,018	$16,606
200%	$4,330	$5084	$6,656	$10,333	$15,921
225%	$3,549	$4,302	$5,875	$9,552	$15,140
250%	$2,671	$3,425	$4,997	$8,674	$14,262
275%	$1,697	$2,450	$4,023	$7,700	$13,288
300%	$626	$1,379	$2,952	$6,629	$12,217
325%	$86	$839	$2,412	$6,089	$11,677
350%	$0	$299	$1,871	$5,548	$11,137
375%	$0	$0	$1,331	$5,008	$10,596
400%	$0	$0	$791	$4,468	$10,056

Source: Kaiser Family Foundation. Health Reform Subsidy Calculator – Premium Assistance for Coverage in Exchanges/Gateways. Available at http://healthreform.kff.org/ SubsidyCalculator.aspx, accessed February 2, 2010.

be to just pass along more of these costs to employees as larger co-payments, deductibles and out-of-pocket costs, often limiting or foregoing wage hikes at the same time.

- A 40 percent tax on high-cost health plans (dubbed the "Cadillac tax") will hit middle-income families hard. These are usually *not* plans with generous benefits, as that term suggests, but instead are plans without basis for their high costs. A recent study found that only 3.7 percent of cost variation could be explained by benefit design or actuarial value—in other words, the policies were virtually no better, just higher cost.[23] Intended to somehow

TABLE 8.2

Health Care Cost Projections For Families Under Senate Health Overhaul Legislation

Annual Income, Family of Four	Cost with Reform Legislation
$36,275 (150% Federal Poverty Line)	Annual Premium: $1,966 Annual Out-of-Pocket Max: $4,200 **Total Risk $6,166** **(17 percent of income)**
$48,367 (200% Federal Poverty Line)	Annual Premium: $3,629 Annual Out-of-Pocket Max $6,300 **Total Risk $9,929** **(21 percent of income)**
$60,458 (250% Federal Poverty Line)	Annual Premium $5,797 Annual Out-of-Pocket Max $6,300 **Total Risk $12,097** **(20 percent of income)**
$72,550 (300% Federal Poverty Line)	Annual Premium: $8,468 Annual Out-of-Pocket Max $8,400 **Total Risk $16,868** **(23 percent of income)**
$84,642 (350% Federal Poverty Line)	Annual Premium: $9,879 Annual Out-of-Pocket Max $8,400 **Total Risk $18,279** **(22 percent of income)**

Source: Kaiser Family Foundation. Health Care Cost Projections for Families under Senate Overhaul Legislation. Available at http://www.kaiserhealthnews.org/

rein in costs, the "Cadillac tax" is a flawed concept—employers will react by trying to limit premiums to avoid the tax while insurers will cut the plans' benefits, thereby again raising cost-sharing to patients. The tax would start in 2013 on plans costing more than $8,500 for individuals and $23,000 for families; by 2016 it would affect 31 million people. Patients with any serious illness or chronic disease will be severely impacted. And to make matters even worse—the Joint Committee on Taxation has reported that revenue from the tax will raise less than 18 percent of the costs of the reform bill. More than 80 percent of tax revenue will come from income taxes paid by employees who had been given pay raises by employers who voluntarily handed over the money they saved by offering health coverage with less benefits![24]

- Many insurers have been aggressively marketing "wellness plans" to employers in recent years. One example is the Healthways SilverSneakers' membership fitness plan provided by many Medicare Advantage plans as a free benefit to seniors around the country.[25] These are private Medicare plans that receive large overpayments, only some of which they allocate to extra benefits (much, of course, goes to profits). This is just another clever way of cherry-picking the market, since it attracts healthier seniors without infirmities that prevent them from participating in these fitness programs. Then, predictably, many insurers charge higher premiums for those not involved in wellness programs. *Market Watch* has reported that insurers already charge policyholders 20 percent more for *not* being involved in wellness programs; this loophole in the new law will allow a 50 percent difference in surcharge.[26]

3. The new bill will fall far short of universal coverage.

Although the new reform bill will likely expand coverage to 32 million people by 2019, much of that expansion will be *under*insurance for reasons described above and because of the many ways by which insurers will split up the risk pool to their advantage. And there will still be more than 23 million Americans without health coverage. That number will be raised further by those choosing to opt out of coverage, either because they are what is called in the industry "Young Invincibles," or many more who cannot afford coverage through an Exchange. The Exchange concept is no panacea. After 15 years of experience, California shut down its Exchange as a failed experiment, having been over-burdened with sicker more costly enrollees and never achieving pricing power.[27]

The reform legislation allocates $5 billion for expansion of state high-risk pools as an aid to people who cannot get coverage due to pre-existing conditions. But here again, these pools have already failed the test of time in more than 30 states, plagued by high premiums, extended waiting lists, and limited benefits while requiring continued funding by state and federal sources.[28] The new federal high-risk pool, which cannot contract with for-profit insurers, will face new challenges in recruiting states to participate and in keeping premiums affordable.[29]

It is already clear that this new high-risk pool is seriously underfunded and will be available to only a small number of uninsured Americans, maximally 7 million and perhaps as few as 200,000 or 3 percent of the target population.[30]

The reform bill will establish four tiers of coverage—from *basic* up to *premium plus*—but it is entirely unclear what services will be covered in each category until a national commission figures that out. What is clear, however, is that the percentage of costs that will be covered—*actuarial value*—will range from as low as 60 or 70 percent in the basic plan for people who obtain coverage through Exchanges. That won't help patients much if they have a significant medical problem. Average costs of hospitalization and care for cardiac bypass surgery today are about $45,000, with hip replacement running about the same. Those costs are certain to be much higher in future years, and will trigger a financial crisis for many families. So how will a patient of modest means with incapacitating hip pain deal with this situation— get a cane and tough it out?

Access to care will further deteriorate as a result of $36 billion in Medicare and Medicaid cuts to safety net hospitals. These hospitals also serve as critical resources for emergency care, kidney dialysis, cancer treatment, mental health care and other services that are too unprofitable for other hospitals to provide. We already hear regularly about more closures of such vital facilities, and the situation will only grow worse with these cuts, adversely impacting not only the uninsured but the tens of millions of underinsured people.

A recent example is the crisis facing St. Vincent's Hospital in Manhattan. After serving its community for more than 150 years, it is now facing bankruptcy for the second time in five years, despite its huge volume—62,000 emergency visits, almost 22,000 hospitalizations, nearly 1,800 births and 263,000 outpatient visits each year. A hospital chain was proposing to take it over, shut down all of its inpatient beds and close out most of its emergency services.[31] That proposal was soon withdrawn, as a firestorm erupted within the community over closure of critical services and the financial opportunism of the for-profit hospital chain.[32]

Although the reconciliation bill did provide an increase in Medicaid reimbursement rates to 100 percent of Medicare payment levels for primary care physicians, that increase is delayed until 2013, and then will last for only two years.[33] Since that temporary increase will likely drop back after that, Medicaid reimbursement will probably remain low. We can expect that a higher proportion of physicians will refuse to see Medicaid patients, leaving patients in even worse straits than they are today.

4. So much change, so little value: It is doubtful that the new bill will significantly improve the quality of care for the U.S. population.

Although the reform bill will make some potentially useful attempts toward improving the quality of care through such means as elimination of cost-sharing requirements for preventive services, establishing a comparative effectiveness research initiative, expansion of health information technology (HIT), and modifications of payment mechanisms (e.g. accountable care organizations (ACOs), and "value modifiers" for physician payments), these are all many years down the road and will be, at best, only incremental tweaks around the edges of the basic problem. The system will still be permeated by perverse incentives that drive a high volume of services, about one-third of which are either inappropriate or unnecessary.[34] Despite limited efforts to strengthen the primary care infrastructure, the system will remain dominated by non-primary care specialties for many years to come, many in oversupply, with little accountability for services rendered.

As noted in earlier chapters, areas of the country with larger numbers of specialists not only have the highest use of medical technologies and the highest health care costs, but also a *lower* quality of care, while areas with more primary care physicians have less use of intensive services, lower costs and a *higher* quality of care.[35,36] One example in cancer care highlights these differences. It has been well documented that patients living in areas with larger numbers of specialists compared to primary care physicians are more likely to have late-stage colorectal cancer when first diagnosed, as well as worse outcomes.[37] That is because primary care is essential to have the best chance for prevention, screening and diagnosis of cancer in early stages. Since the new health care legislation does little to improve the ratio of primary care physicians to the general population, our physician workforce will likely remain top-heavy in specialists.

These are some of the factors that call into question whether this version of health care reform can actually improve the system's quality of care:

- *Expected increase in cost-sharing (meaning the employee pays more than before) as employers downgrade the actuarial value of their coverage and as insurers market their underinsurance products in the individual market and through Exchanges.* It has been well documented that the higher co-payments and deductibles lead many patients to delay or even forego necessary care, leading to later diagnosis of more complicated disease and worse outcomes. The original intent of cost-sharing was to reduce health care costs by forcing patients to be more responsible and judicious in their health-seeking behaviors (moral hazard). But that theory has been largely discredited. It has become clear that greater financial barriers to initial care lead patients to forego preventive services and early care for new illnesses. This delay results in later diagnosis of more complicated and costly problems. And the outcomes are worse.[38,39] A just-published study of Medicare Advantage plans puts numbers on this issue. Plans that increased co-payments for primary care by 95 percent and 74 percent for specialty care documented these results: fewer outpatient visits, more hospital admissions, and longer hospital stays, with greater impacts on patients with hypertension, diabetes or a history of acute myocardial infarction.[40]
- *Critical shortage of primary care physicians and underfunded primary care infrastructure.* As is well known, a majority of physicians in many parts of the country will not see patients on Medicaid because of low reimbursement that often does not even cover their overhead costs in seeing these patients. In view of federal and state deficits, we can anticipate that the present crisis in access to care for these patients will only get worse as states progressively cut back on benefits and as reimbursement rates remain low.
- *Expanded use of new information technologies, such as electronic medical records, is likely to be disappointing in terms of its potential to improve outcomes of care for the population.* There is no doubt that computerized systems can improve the quality of care in integrated systems, such as the Veterans Administration, Kaiser Permanente and Group Health

Cooperative. But this does not hold in the larger for-profit, non-integrated parts of the delivery system. We can predict that there will be less potential for information technology to improve care because of other important factors, such as financial barriers to care and other factors leading to health care disparities. There is also a growing body of literature indicating that increased reliance on computerized records to improve quality outcomes, by itself, is not a silver bullet. Much of the growing use of medical computing has been driven by financial and billing reasons, not quality of care. And quality improvement efforts usually involve *process* measures (such as use of beta blockers after a heart attack or use of hemoglobin A1C in diabetes), which are often not good measures of actual outcomes.[41,42]

5. Insurance "reforms" are incomplete and will be largely ineffective.

As we have seen, the insurance industry's gamble on health care reform was to give up some of its practices, such as using pre-existing conditions as a reason to deny coverage, in return for government subsidies that may facilitate expansion of the insured population by up to 32 million by 2019. But it would be an illusion to think that medical underwriting and the ability of insurers to still cherry-pick the market will become a thing of the past. The reform bill is very friendly to the insurance industry, as these examples show:[43]

- Retention of the anti-trust exemption for insurers
- Overpayments to Medicare Advantage (MA) programs are not actually eliminated; instead, a new "competitive bidding" approach will be substituted; in 2014, MA plans will be required to have MLRs of 85 percent, but those levels can readily be gamed lower. A recent analysis of future MA payments funded by the Commonwealth Fund found that some areas of the country will receive extra payments up to 17 percent of Medicare fee-for-service costs, while other areas will be paid about 6 percent less than those costs.[44]
- Elimination of pre-existing conditions as a way to deny coverage is delayed until 2014; even then, all existing employer-sponsored (ESI) plans will be grandfathered in without coverage reforms.

- Insurers can still hike premiums by a 3:1 ratio for age and 1.5:1 for smokers.
- Medical loss ratios (MLRs) can be set as low as 80 percent in the individual market and 85 percent for ESI plans; actuarial values for basic coverage (whatever that will come to mean!) can be set as low as 60 percent, and insurers will have many opportunities to game the system by counting other costs against patient care, such as disease management, wellness and information management programs.
- Creation of a "Young Invincibles" policy for young adults less than 30 years of age with an initial annual deductible of $5,950 (indexed over time).
- Annual caps, maximum amounts that insurance companies must pay out in a given year, will not be prohibited until 2014;[45] all existing plans will be exempted permanently from either annual or lifetime caps.[46]
- Elimination of the public option.
- Even in more regulated states, insurers will still be in charge of coverage policies, and are likely to design low-benefit plans for healthier enrollees.
- Exchanges are delayed until 2014, and then are only available to the uninsured and *some* employees of small employers, but not to the large majority of insured people, regardless of their desire to change plans.
- Insurers are permitted to sell their plans across state lines, an approach long exploited by many insurers whereby they can select states with lax insurance regulations. Since they are subject only to the regulations of the state they are headquartered in, they can thereby avoid more rigorous regulations in other states.[47]

Insurers clearly won the political battle over reform. Here is how Robert Reich, Professor of Public Policy at the University of California Berkeley, has summarized this outcome:

> "From the start, opponents of the public option have wanted to portray it as a big government preying upon the market, and private insurers as the embodiment of the market. But it's just

the reverse. Private insurers are exempt from competition. As a result, they are becoming ever more powerful. And it's not just their economic power that's worrying. It's also their political power, as we've learned over the last ten months. Economic and political power is a potent combination. Without some mechanism forcing private insurers to compete, we're going to end up with a national healthcare system that's controlled by a handful of very large corporations accountable neither to American voters nor to the market."[48]

6. Health care "reform" will add immeasurably to the cost and waste of new layers of bureaucracy without added value.

Just think of all the new layers of bureaucracy that will be added to our already woefully cumbersome system. Implementing and maintaining the increased fragmentation of financing health care will become an administrative nightmare. And much of that effort is just to bail out a dying insurance industry that would fail without government subsidies and protection. Taxpayers are being asked to pay the continuing high cost of government subsidies for an expanded and very expensive private insurance bureaucracy, allowing it to keep marketing its underinsurance products while its administrative overhead is typically eight or ten times the cost of traditional Medicare.[49]

The new reform law will require many additional layers of bureaucracy, each with its own attendant increased costs. The Internal Revenue Service will add new staff to police the individual mandate and fine people who don't buy insurance, for which $5 to $10 billion are allocated. The multi-payer financing system will remain an administrative monster. Based on the experience in Massachusetts over the last several years, administrative costs for running the Exchanges are expected to run about 4 percent of premium costs. And many key questions remain to be answered as to how the law will be implemented, ranging from definition of essential benefits, which 1,300 private insurers are required to cover, to whether and how standardized claims forms can be developed.

Overall assessment

In view of the many drawbacks to the new reform legislation, despite some of its benefits, how can we sum up what we will get? This insightful observation cuts to the heart of the matter:

Dr. Marcia Angell, former editor of the *New England Journal of Medicine* and author of the excellent book, *The Truth about the Drug Companies, and What To Do About It*, makes this important point, reminding us that the political discourse has focused mainly on *government* spending on health care, completely missing the point of what *we as patients and families* will be forced to pay:

> "The reform bill wrongly retains the central role of the private insurance companies and requires millions of people to buy their products at whatever price they charge. True, some of the industry's discriminatory practices will be outlawed, but if that adds to their costs, they can simply raise premiums. The pharmaceutical industry can also continue to charge whatever it likes. If the bill is fully implemented (which I doubt), it may restrain the growth of government health spending, which is all the CBO cares about. Obama knows that a single payer system is the only way to provide universal care while controlling costs, but he is unwilling to throw his weight behind it. All he seems to want now is the political victory of getting a health bill passed—any bill, no matter how untenable."[50]

MULTI-PAYER VS. SINGLE PAYER FINANCING: A NO-BRAINER

The absurdity of market proponents' claims, repeatedly espousing the supposed greater "efficiencies" of the free market and warning us against the threat of a "government takeover" of health care, could not be more obvious. Competition in open markets may work well in other areas of the economy, but it doesn't apply in health care, where industries are consolidated and hold the upper hand in setting prices, while patients and their families as consumers have restricted choice and very little bargaining power. Many examples of this power differential have been discussed in this book.

As a result of the new health care law, the private insurance marketplace will become even more complex and intrusive than it is now concerning the everyday needs of patients and the practices of their physicians. The main bureaucrats separating patients and physicians from needed health care today and in the future are *private*, not public.

And continuation of private financing foregoes some $400 billion a year in cost savings when compared to the efficiencies of a not-for-profit public single payer system like Medicare.

Here is what we will have when we put single payer in place. The major differences between what we have now and what can be achieved by not-for-profit public financing, coupled with a private delivery system, are shown in Table 8.3.

Medicare is not a perfect program, and has been subjected to many pressures to privatize over its history that have raised problems of cost, and sometimes even of access and quality. These problems include lack of an adequate system to make coverage decisions based on scientific evidence, wide disparities in reimbursement patterns from one part of the country to another, overutilization of inappropriate and unnecessary care, variable quality of care, and fraud among some providers. These problems have been described in my earlier book, *Shredding the Social Contract: The Privatization of Medicare.*[51] In spite of its problems, however, Medicare is rated higher by patients compared to private coverage, whether for access, costs or quality.[52] Moreover, Medicare is managed with an administrative overhead of just 3 percent compared to overhead costs of 18 to 20 percent for commercial carriers and 26.5 percent for investor-owned Blues.[53] A 2005 study found that 22 percent of private insurer premiums go to sales, marketing, billing and other administrative tasks (often to deny claims or coverage!), all of which are unnecessary in a publicly-financed program.[54]

So single payer based on improved Medicare is an excellent model upon which to build real health care reform. We will return to this approach in more detail in Chapter 11, but for now we need to move to the next chapter to consider what lessons we can learn from the

TABLE 8.3

A Superior System: Single Payer Bill vs. Reconciliation Bill

Single Payer

Universal Coverage..............Yes Everyone is covered automatically from birth.

Full Range of Benefits..........Yes Coverage for all necessary services.

Cost Containment...............Yes Large scale cost controls (negotiated fee schedule with physicians, bulk purchasing of drugs, hospital budgeting, capital planning, etc.) ensure that benefits are sustainable over the long term.

Affordability......................Yes Costs are kept affordable by spreading risk across one large risk pool, more than 300 million Americans, by shifting to a not-for-profit system, and by reining in waste and unnecessary care.

Choice of Doctor & Hospital..Yes Patients have full choice of their doctor and hospital, none of them being "out-of-network".

Improved Quality of Care ......Yes Through universal access to all necessary care: prevention, early diagnosis, evidence-based treatments, & rehabilitative care.

More Equitable ....Yes Health disparities are reduced. Health care becomes a right based on medical need, not a commodity based on ability to pay.

Savings ....Yes Redirects about $400 billion in administrative waste to patient care; no net increase in health spending.

Progressive Financing..........Yes Premiums & out-of-pocket costs are replaced with a progressive income distribution. 95% of Americans pay less than they are now.

Sustainability....................Yes Not-for-profit public financing, coupled with a more accountable private delivery system, can reduce bureaucracy and provide necessary health care to our entire population for generations to come.

Source: Adapted with permission from Himmelstein, DU, Woolhandler, S and Physicians for a National Health Program

TABLE 8.3 (continued)

A Superior System: Single Payer Bill vs. Reconciliation Bill

Reconciliation Bill

Universal Coverage	No	More than 23 million Americans are projected to remain uninsured in 2019 while tens of millions are underinsured.
Full Range of Benefits	No	Insurers continue to strip-down policies and increase patients' co-payments and deductibles (e.g. a policy with a $2,000 deductible and 20 percent co-insurance for the next $15,000 of care).
Cost Containment	No	Uncontrolled costs will ensure that any gains in coverage are quickly erased as government is forced to hike spending or slash benefits.
Affordability	No	Tens of millions of middle-class Americans will be pressured to buy defective insurance policies covering only 70 percent of health care costs at premium costs up to 9.5 percent of their annual income.
Choice of Doctor & Hospital	No	Insurance companies will continue to deny and limit care and to maintain restrictive, often changing networks.
Improved Quality of Care	Uncertain	But probably not, in view of limits to access based on skyrocketing costs of care.
More Equitable	No	Increasing gap between haves and have nots; access to care under expanded Medicaid will be limited because of low reimbursement in an underfunded program.
Savings	No	Increases health spending by about $1 trillion over ten years. Adds further layers of administrative bloat to our health system through the introduction of state-based Exchanges.
Progressive Financing	No	Continues the unfair financing of health care whereby costs are disproportionately paid by middle- and lower-income Americans and those families facing acute or chronic illness.
Sustainability	No	Will result in runaway health care costs— a bonanza for health care markets; Medicare cuts may not be politically feasible as a means to pay for the bill; state and federal governments will be hard-pressed to maintain adequate funding.

legislative train wreck of 2009-2010 over health care.

References

1. Himmelstein, DU, Woolhandler, S. Obama's reform: No cure for what ails us. *British Medical Journal*, March 30, 2010.
2. Hamsher, J. Fact sheet: The truth about the health care bill. FireDogLake, March 19, 2010.
3. Galewitz, P. Plastic surgeons cry foul over 'Botax' proposal in Senate health bill. *Kaiser Health News*, November 20, 2009.
4. Rockoff, JD. Knives drawn over 'Botax'. *Wall Street Journal*, December 4, 2009:A3.
5. Russell, L. Preventing chronic disease: An important investment, but don't count on cost savings. *Health Affairs* 28(1): 42-5, 2009.
6. Sidorov, J. It ain't necessarily so: The electronic health record and the unlikely prospect of reducing health care costs. *Health Aff (Millwood)* 25 (4):1179-85, 2006.
7. Austin, DA, Hungerford, TL. *The Market Structure of the Health Insurance Industry*. Washington, D.C. Congressional Research Service, November 17, 2009.
8. Ladapo, JA, Horwitz, JR, Weinstein, MC, Gazelle, S, Cutler, DM. Adoption and spread of new imaging technology: A case study. *Health Affairs* 28(6): w1122-32, 2009.
9. Kaiser Health News staff. True or false: Seven concerns about the new health law, March 31, 2010.
10. Kolata, G. Law may do little to help curb unnecessary care. *New York Times,* March 30, 2010: D1.
11. Press release. AFGE Statement on FEHBP 2010 premium increase. Washington, D.C. American Federation of Government Employees. September 29, 2009.
12. Graham Center One-Pager. Who will have health insurance in 2025? Washington, D.C. The Robert Graham Center. Policy Studies in Family Medicine and Primary Care. *Am Fam Physician* 72 (10): 1989, 2005.
13. Fein, O, Himmelstein, DU, Woolhandler, S. Press release. Chicago, Il. Physicians for a National Health Program. December 22, 2009.
14. Pear, R. Expanding health coverage and shoring up Medicare: Is it double-counting? *New York Times,* December 29, 2009: A18.
15. Samuelson, R. Get real on health costs: Obama's plan won't cut spending. *Business Week*, December 21, 2009: 36.
16. Office of the Actuary, Centers for Medicare and Medicaid Services. Health spending projections through 2019: The recession's impact continues. *Health Affairs*, February 4, 2010.
17. Wuerker, M. Political Cartoon: Rock the Boat. *Kaiser Health News*, December 10, 2009.
18. CBO. The health care law. Questioning the cost of the health care overhaul,

April 3, 2010: A11.

19. Kaiser Family Foundation. Health Reform Subsidy Calculator – Premium Assistance for Coverage in Exchanges/Gateways. Available at http://healthreform.kff.org/SubsidyCalculator.aspx, accessed February 2, 2010.

20. Schoen, C, Doty, M, Collins, SR, Holmgren, AL. Commonwealth Fund, Insured but not protected: How many adults are underinsured, the experiences of adults with inadequate coverage mirror those of their uninsured peers. *Health Affairs Web Exclusive*, June 14, 2005.

21. Kaiser Family Foundation. Health Care Cost Projections for Families under Senate Overhaul Legislation. Available at http://www.kaiserhealthnews.org/

22. Jost, T. The health care reform reconciliation bill (updated). Blog. Timothy Jost, March 19, 2010.

23. Gabel, J, Pickreign, J, McDevitt, R, Briggs, T. Taxing Cadillac plans may produce Chevy results. *Health Aff*, on-line, December 3, 2009.

24. Herbert, B. OpEd. A less than honest policy. *New York Times*, December 29, 2009.

25. Blue Shield of California. Blue Shield of California to offer award-winning fitness program to Medicare beneficiaries in San Bernardino. January 18, 2010.

26. Britt, R. Experts: Critical loophole in Senate health bill. *Market Watch*. January 7, 2010.

27. Building a National Insurance Exchange: Lessons from California. Issue Brief. California HealthCare Foundation, July 2009.

28. American Diabetes Association. High-risk pools. Health Insurance Resource Manual. Alexandria, VA, 2006.

29. Mathews, AW. High-risk health pool faces start-up problems. *Wall Street Journal*, March 27-28, 2010: A4.

30. Merlis, M. Health coverage for the high-risk uninsured: Policy options for design of the temporary high-risk pool. National Institute for Health Care Reform, May 27, 2010.

31. Hartocollis, A. Critical care: The fall of St. Vincent's in Manhattan. *New York Times*, February 3, 2010: A20.

32. Hartocollis, A. Hospital network that made offer to take over St. Vincents withdraws it. *New York Times*, February 5, 2010: A18.

33. Ibid # 22.

34. Wennberg, JB, Fisher, ES, Skinner, JS. Geography and the debate over Medicare reform. *Health Affairs Web Exclusive* W-103, February 13, 2002.

35. Fisher, ES, Welch, HG. Avoiding the unintended consequences of growth in medical care: How might more be worse? *JAMA* 281: 446-53, 1999.

36. Parchman, M, Culter, S. Primary care physicians and avoidable hospitatlization. J Fam Pract 39: 123-6, 1994.

37. Roetzheim, RG, Pal, N, Gonzalez, EC et al. The effects of physician supply on the early detection of colorectal cancer. *J Fam Pract* 48 (11): 850-8, 1999.

38. Nyman, J. Is moral hazard inefficient? The policy implications of a new theory. *Health Aff (Millwood)* 23 (5):194-99, 2004.

39. Geyman, JP. Moral hazard and consumer-directed health care: A fundamentally

flawed concept. *Intl J Health Serv* 37 (2): 333-51, 2007.

40. Trivedi, AN, Moloo, H, Mor, V. Increased ambulatory care copayments and hospitalizations among the elderly. *N Engl J Med* 362(4): 320-8. 2010.

41. Chaudhry, B, Wang, J, Wu, S, Maglione, M, Mojica, W et al. Systematic review: Impact of health information technology on quality, efficiency and costs of medical care. *Ann Int Med* 144 (10): 742-52, 2006.

42. Himmelstein, DU, Wright, A, Woolhandler, S. Hospital computing and the costs and quality of care: A national study. *Amer J Med* 123 (1): 40-6, 2010.

43. Tri-Committee House Staff. House-Senate Comparison of Key Provisions. December 29, 2009.

44. Biles, B, Arnold, G. Medicare Advantage payment provisions in the Health Care and Education Affordability Reconciliation Act (H.R. 4872). Washington, D.C. George Washington University. School of Public Health and Health Services. March 26, 2010.

45. Sharp, D. Maine widow celebrates law ending insurance caps. Bloomberg Businessweek, April 26, 2010.

46. Andrews, M. Caps on coverage. A big point of conflict. *New York Times*, January 27, 2010: A15.

47.   Hall, M. The geography of health insurance regulation: A guide to identifying, exploiting, and policing market boundaries. *Health Aff (Millwood)* 19 (2): 173-82, 2000.

48. Reich, R. Meet your new health insurance overlords. *The Progressive Populist* 16 (1); p.15, January 1-15, 2010.

49. Committee on Energy and Commerce. New report highlights Medicare Advantage insurers' higher administrative spending. Washington, D.C. December 9, 2009.

50. Angell, M. Obama at one. A National Forum. *The Nation* 290(4): 17-8, 2010.

51. Geyman, JP. *Shredding the Social Contract: The Privatization of Medicare.* Monroe, ME. Common Courage Press, 2006.

52. Davis, K, Schoen, C, Doty, M, Tenney, K. Medicare vs. private insurance: Rhetoric and reality. Health Affairs Web Exclusive W21, October 9, 2002.

53. Himmelstein, DU. The National Health Program Slide-Show Guide. Center for National Health Program Studies. Cambridge, MA, 2000.

54. Kahn, JG, Kronick, R, Kryer, M, Gans, DN. The cost of health insurance administration in California: Estimates for insurers, physicians, and hospitals. *Health Affairs (Millwood)* 24 (6): 1629-39, 2005.

CHAPTER 9

Wall Street Wins, Main Street Loses:
Lessons from this Legislative Train Wreck

"Politics is the conduct of public affairs for private advantage...
Reform is a thing that mostly satisfies reformers opposed to
reformation."
>— Ambrose Bierce (1842-1914?), American editorialist,
> journalist and author of *The Devil's Dictionary*

"Markets reduce everything, including human beings (labor) and
nature (land), to commodities. We have a market economy but
we cannot have a market society."
>— George Soros, billionaire investor
> and author of *The Capitalist Threat*[1]

As we saw in the last chapter, this latest massive effort to reform our
health care system, despite all the hyperbole of its historic significance,
has missed the key target objectives. Future years will prove it to
be a very expensive failure in reining in health care costs, making
necessary care affordable for the population, and improving the quality
of care. Instead, many new layers of bureaucracy will be added to our
already cumbersome system. As corporate stakeholders in the medical-
industrial complex reap their rewards, the health care needs of ordinary
Americans will be sacrificed to their unearned profits. Wall Street wins,
Main Street loses.

What take-away lessons can we learn from this health policy
disaster so as to do better when we inevitably try again? That is the
focus of this chapter.

THE MAJOR LESSONS FROM THE REFORM EFFORT

There are many reasons for this reform attempt going off the tracks.
They can be categorized in different ways, but these seem to me to

capture the most important ones. They are all interrelated, and stem from economic, social, political, cultural and historic factors. And we can't avoid a sense of *déjà vu* comparing the lessons from this most recent reform attempt with those over the last 100 years.

1. Framing of issues and the entire political process were hijacked by the very interests that are largely responsible for systemic problems of health care.

As discussed in Chapter 3, stakeholders in the medical industrial complex were actively involved in shaping the issues and guiding the political process from the beginning. They are expert at promoting their own interests through many means, including campaign contributions to their elected representatives (particularly those in pivotal policy-making positions); rotating allies through the revolving door between industry, government and the K Street lobbying nexus; advertising campaigns through disease advocacy groups, Astroturf organizations and similar groups; and influencing how the media report on the health care debate.

Despite claims by its supporters that health care reform 2010 is a great advance comparable to programs of the Great Society, this legislation is really more conservative than it might appear. As Robert Reich points out: "Don't believe anyone who says Obama's health care legislation marks a swing of the pendulum back toward the Great Society and the New Deal. Obama's health bill is a very conservative piece of legislation, building on a Republican rather than a New Deal foundation."[2] Both the individual and employer mandates were Republican ideas and proposals in the 1990s, while President Nixon proposed an employer mandate in the early 1970s.[3,4]

Here are some of the ways in which the issues were incorrectly framed from the start:

- "We should build on our existing system, not fundamentally change it" (thereby disregarding our long history of failed incremental reforms, avoiding dealing with system problems in new ways, and neglecting the findings of many public opinion polls that have shown that a large portion of the public believe fundamental reform is required).
- Basic questions were never asked, such as: Should health care be a right available to everyone based on medical need or a privilege

based on ability to pay?; should health care be a for-profit commodity for sale on an open market or a public utility like fire and police protection?; is employer-sponsored health insurance stable enough to build upon?; should we bail out a dying private health insurance industry through government subsidies?; and what are the real drivers of unsustainable inflation of health care costs?

• Discussions of the failures of the market were not addressed; instead market interests kept telling us that markets can fix our system's problems, an assertion never questioned by the media.

As a predictable result of this misguided framing, the full scope of policy alternatives was never fleshed out, single payer financing was never put on the table, cost containment and reimbursement issues were not effectively addressed, and corporate stakeholders were allowed to dictate to their own advantage many of the provisions of the final health care bills in Congress.

2. The democratic process was commandered by corporations.

We weren't blindsided by the poor outcome of this year's reform process. It was predictable from the start. The Obama Administration made the same mistake as the Clinton Administration by inviting the major corporate stakeholders to the negotiating table, assuming that consensus there would bring reform. Those stakeholders that offered "pledges" made gestures of support for "reform" that would secure large new markets for themselves. The "alliance" for reform was never one in fact, as became evident in the later stages of the debate when they began fighting against each other, sometimes even within themselves.

We saw a failure of leadership at all governing levels, including the White House, the Senate and the House. As with other major problems, such as the meltdown of the financial industry, President Obama was all too cautious about the task. He surrounded himself with advisors who were insiders in health care industries that are part of the problem. As an example, White House Director of the Office of Health Reform Nancy-Ann DeParle received more than $6 million while serving on boards of directors of at least half a dozen companies that were targets of federal investigations, whistleblower lawsuits, and other regulatory actions.[5] A much better choice would have been Wendell Potter, whistle-blower against the industry he served for some 25 years!

Then Obama flip-flopped on key issues, such as the public option, and tossed the reform process to Congress "to work out the details." The feeding frenzy was on. As we saw in Chapter 2, Elizabeth Fowler, an insurance industry representative turned Senate staffer, largely wrote the Senate Finance Committee's bill, while successful lobbyists found their verbatim words put out as press statements by legislators whom they had targeted.[6] By the time the health care reform law was finally passed, the lobbying industry had reaped its own bonanza—about 1,750 businesses and organizations had hired some 4,525 lobbyists— eight for every member of Congress, at a cost of $1.2 billion.[7]

This entire scenario has lengthy historical roots. In a recent article, Henry Giroux, who holds the Global TV Network Chair Professorship at Canada's McMaster University in the English and Cultural Studies Department, traces the triumph of corporate sovereignty over the democratic process in the U.S. over the last three decades. Here's how he sums it up:

> "For over 30 years, the American public has been reared on a neoliberal dystopian vision that legitimates itself through the largely unchallenged claim that there are no alternatives to a market-driven society, that economic growth should not be constrained by considerations of social costs or moral responsibility and that democracy and capitalism were virtually synonymous. At the heart of this market rationality is an egocentric philosophy and culture of cruelty that sold off public goods and services to the highest bidders in the corporate and private sectors, while simultaneously dismantling those public spheres, social protections and institutions serving the public good. As economic power freed itself from traditional government regulations, a new global financial class reasserted the prerogatives of capital and systemically destroyed those public spheres advocating social equality and an educated citizenry as a condition for a viable democracy. At the same time, economic deregulation merged powerfully with the ideology of individual responsibility, effectively evading any notion of corporate accountability to a broader public."[8]

3. The quest for bipartisanship was futile; reform got run over in the middle of the road.

Answers to the fundamental questions about the future of U.S. health care, such as roles of the market vs. the government and health care as a right vs. a privilege, cannot be found in the middle of the road. They are closer to polar opposites. Public financing of health care should have been the option on the left (Medicare for All) vs. the right's limited government, social Darwinism approach. Instead, our political leadership sought a so-called centrist approach under the banner of bipartisanship, thereby compromising meaningful reform and relegating it to failure. The logical disconnects within the centrist approach boggle the mind, by allowing a "reform" proposal, for example, to require individuals to purchase inadequate private health insurance while disallowing any regulation of insurance premiums. Reflecting on President Obama's health care address to Congress in September, Rabbi Michael Lerner, editor of *Tikkun Magazine*, had this to say:

> "The confusion, for once, is not with the media but with the incoherence of a centrist politics. Obama wishes to relieve the suffering of Americans, but he does not wish to challenge the profit-over-everything old "Bottom Line" of the competitive marketplace. Unfortunately for him and for most Americans, he can't have it both ways. FDR recognized that—and so was willing to stand up to the vested interests of the class from which he emerged, not only rhetorically, as Obama is willing to do at some rare moments like his Health Care speech, but in the actual policies he promoted."[9]

Beyond logic and internal consistency, however, the centrist approach failed in political terms anyway. After months of trying to appease the GOP in Congress by many compromises, Republicans ended up voting in a unified block against reform bills brought by Democrats to committee or floor votes. And even as they did so, they would not acknowledge that the plans they were vigorously opposing were concepts that they had promoted some years earlier! Republican proposals for employer and individual mandates in past years illustrate this point, since Republicans took a united stand against them in this last round of bills.[10,11]

4. Market failure was not recognized as the wellspring of our problems.

The early commitment made to build on our present system meant the retention of multi-payer financing, preservation and nurturing of our market-based system, and acceptance of the myth that "competition" in health care markets can rein in costs. Despite all the contortions by legislators and policy makers to give an illusion of cost controls, we overlooked our experience of recent decades—markets don't work in health care as they do in other parts of the economy, and the public's need to contain costs flies in the face of corporate stakeholders' drives for increased revenues. This business as usual approach was ordained to fail. By trying to gain the support and agreement of market stakeholders, policymakers were looking for reform in all the wrong places.

Instead of cost containment and affordable access to care, here is what we can expect now that the politicians have finished crafting their illusion of reform:

- Widespread underinsurance, with high deductibles, co-payments and out-of-network costs, rising premiums, and coverage requirements as low as 60 percent of health care costs.
- Further gaming of the insurance industry to cherry pick the "new" system.
- Departure from the market of many private Medicare Advantage plans; Humana, as the biggest player in that market with revenue gains from public programs increasing from $271 million in 2008 to $474 million in 2009, is already eying more lucrative markets in management of specialty biotech drugs and chronic disease management programs.[12]
- Continuous escalation of prices by drug and medical device manufacturers, hospitals, physicians, and other members of the medical industrial complex.
- Persistent core group of at least 23 million Americans without insurance.
- *Reduced* choice of health plans, physicians and hospitals.
- Any "savings" from Medicare cuts or taxes on stakeholders resulting in passing on those costs to consumers, thereby driving their out-of-pocket costs even higher.
- Increased tiering of care, with many millions of Americans still

unable to afford necessary care, delaying care and suffering the consequences—more morbidity and increasing numbers of preventable deaths.

5. The private health insurance industry is in a death spiral, and does not provide enough value to justify a bailout.

Policymakers, legislators, and almost all of the corporate media have been complicit in bailing out a dying industry. The new health care "reform" bill extends its life for a few more years by imposing individual and employer mandates with generous subsidies to help many millions of Americans buy the industry's defective products. But the writing is on the wall—the industry has abused the public trust for too many years, does not offer enough value to survive, and has already become dependent on government subsidies through tax benefits and subsidized public programs (i.e. Medicare Advantage and privatized Medicaid programs).

The impending death of private health insurance as we know it in this country has been recognized for some years as inevitable. Here is what Bruce Bodaken, CEO of Blue Shield of California, had to say in 2005:

> "The state's private-sector health care market is in deep trouble and could implode unless all the players collaborate to provide coverage for the uninsured and reduce costs that are sending premiums skyward. Without action to overcome the problems of cost and access, the market will get to the point where the balance of power will move from the private market to the halls of government. And when that happens, it's hard to know what the solution coming out the door will look like."[13]

More recently, when this matter was discussed at a large meeting of health economists at the Federal Reserve Bank of Chicago, the unquestioned consensus among participants was that the insurance industry no longer offers enough value to survive.[14]

As discussed in detail in my 2009 book, *Do Not Resuscitate: Why the Health Insurance Industry is Dying, and How We Must Replace It*, these are the major reasons why the industry is on a death march:

- uncontrolled inflation of health care costs
- growing unaffordability of premiums and health care
- decreasing levels of insurance coverage
- growing economic insecurity and hardship, even for the insured
- fragmentation and inefficiency
- shrinking private insurance markets
- adverse selection in shrinking risk pools
- cutbacks in government subsidies for privatized public programs[15]

Two current examples illustrate how the death spiral works by adverse selection in shrinking markets. In California, Anthem Blue Cross, a Wellpoint subsidiary, has a stranglehold over the individual market. Its recent attempt to hike premiums by up to 39 percent was defended by the company as necessary because of rising costs of care. The reasons for this dynamic are clear: as more people drop coverage because of costs, the insurer is left with sicker enrollees, thereby decreasing its profitability. As fewer enrollees lead to higher premiums, the vicious cycle feeds on itself.[16] In Massachusetts, where a law was enacted in 2006 much along the lines of the 2010 federal law, many young and healthy people are gaming the individual mandate by signing up for Blue Cross Blue Shield coverage for three months or less, getting such pricey care as fertility treatments or knee surgery, then dropping the coverage and paying the state's minimal penalty of $93 for not having insurance. That of course drives up costs and premiums for other people and small businesses.[17]

Even as Anthem Blue Cross hikes its premiums and cuts coverage in California, it continues to violate state laws and regulations in many areas. The California Department of Managed Health Care (DMHC) has issued 475 enforcement actions against the company over the last ten years, 275 of which have been levied since early 2009.[18]

While some in this country call for more regulation of the industry as the way forward, pointing to the experience of some countries in Western Europe, the industry has successfully worked its way around regulators at both state and federal levels. Moreover, we have seen how the industry fought off serious threats in this new "reform" law, such as retention of its anti-trust exemption, killing off the public option and avoidance of federal rate-setting powers. In the Dutch and Swiss systems, insurers are heavily regulated, including requirements for community-rated premiums that are uniform for all ages of enrollees.[19] The industry in this country would never accept that level of regulation without going out of business altogether.

6. The Obama Administration has not been willing to confront the special interests and address the real problems.

While conveniently denying that unfettered health care markets were the problem and listening to their advocates that they would help fix our problems, the real problems requiring fundamental reform—soaring costs, unaffordability, inadequate access, and mediocre quality of care—fell by the wayside. Instead the debate was distracted by details, where many of the "solutions" worked in opposite directions from these basic problems. What would be agreeable to market stakeholders became the question, not what would meet the needs of our population. As stakeholders and their lobbyists worked their magic behind the scenes, we ended up with a law without price controls, without reimbursement reform (just studies or pilot projects years down the road), without limits on volume of excessive care, and with a powerless future Center for Comparative Effectiveness Research. In his excellent recent book, *Empire of Illusion: The End of Literacy and the Triumph of Spectacle*, Chris Hedges, for many years a foreign correspondent for the *New York Times* and now a senior fellow at The Nation Institute, gives us this perspective:

> "The attempt to create a health-care plan that also conciliates the corporations that profit from the misery and illnesses of tens of millions of Americans is naïve, at best, and probably disingenuous. This conciliation insists that we can coax these corporations, which are listed on the stock exchange and exist to maximize profit, to transform themselves into social-service agencies that will provide adequate health care for all Americans."[20]

Another broader perspective on why we are unable to confront the reality of our present and future problems is offered by Jeff Faux, political scientist, founder and distinguished fellow at the Economic Policy Institute:

> "Obama's now obvious deficiencies as a fighter for the causes he eloquently expounds… is imbedded in a system of governance

that for the last three decades has been incapable of dealing with the future because its most important financiers are still profiting from the present."[21]

Denial went further—under the banner of U.S. exceptionalism, we ignored the experience of other industrialized countries that have dealt with these problems more effectively than we have. It was further denied that all incremental attempts to reform our market-based system have already failed. Our political leaders were unwilling to consider well-documented findings of health policy science that could lead us out of our morass.

As an admitted pragmatic centrist, Obama cannot claim the moral authority of principled leadership. Recall his impassioned speech to a labor group during his 2003 campaign in Illinois on the urgent need for single payer universal coverage (Chapter 3, p. 63). Instead of taking on the powers, he surrendered in advance. Compare that with the courageous presidential leadership of FDR during his 1936 campaign:

> "We know now that Government by organized money is just as dangerous as Government by organized mob. The old enemies of peace—business and financial monopoly, speculation, reckless banking, class antagonism, sectionalism, war profiteering... [these interests] had begun to consider the Government of the United States as a mere appendage to their own affairs... They are unanimous in hate for me, and I welcome their hatred. I should have it said of my first Administration that in it the forces of selfishness and of lust for power met their match. I should have it said of my second Administration that in it these forces met their master."[22]

7. Real reform was labeled "politically infeasible;" the "reform" we got, while politically feasible, will fail.

The Obama Administration fell into the same trap that ensnared the Clinton Administration 15 years earlier—they both dismissed the single payer financing option as politically infeasible from the get-go. And as the political process went forward, the predictable result was that stakeholders got their way and real reform went by the wayside. Consider these similarities:

The Clinton Health Plan (CHP), a 1,342-page bill, died in Congress in 1994 (without even a floor vote) after being picked apart by warring interest groups. Colin Gordon, historian at the University of Iowa, described the politics in this way:

> "The CHP's fatal flaw, at least in these terms, lay in its attempt to combine employer mandates (which attracted health interests and repelled many employers) and cost control (which attracted employers and repelled health interests). This pairing made for a slow dance to the right, as reaction set in from all quarters against employer mandates, against spending controls, against any increased federal presence in health care. This reaction showed up, in turn, in the whining of Congressional conservatives, the CHP's drastic revision by Democrats, the various (misnamed) 'mainstream' or 'moderate' alternatives, and the final admission by Congressional leaders that they had nothing left to pass."[23]

In 2009-2010, we witnessed the same process of waning support by initial "supporters," with increasingly powerful opposition by special interests divided among, and often within, themselves. Thus, employers rejected mandates and feared increased taxes; unions feared loss of benefits and rising premiums; hospitals and physicians feared Medicare cuts; insurers feared erosion of the individual mandate even though they had avoided rate controls of their premiums; Democrats fought among themselves as a flawed legislative package cost too much; and much of the public became more concerned that system "reform" wouldn't help them.

8. Senate "rules" block the democratic process.

Parliamentary self-imposed rules in the Senate that allow 41 out of 100 voting senators to indefinitely extend debate and prevent a final floor vote on a bill—a filibuster—have become commonplace. As we saw in the previous chapter, the Senate health care bill was delayed by 25 days in a filibuster, second only to the 26 day stalling action imposed by anti-war legislators in 1917 over a measure allowing the arming of merchant ships during World War I.[24]

Filibusters used to be the exception. In the 1960s, they affected only about 8 percent of major legislation. That number increased to 27 percent in the 1980s and ballooned to 70 percent after 2006, when the

Republicans lost their majority in the Senate.[25] That big change in our governance has taken place with little coverage by the corporate media and no real public debate.

The implications of this change bodes ill for the democratic process. The 40 Republican senators (before the election of Scott Brown in Massachusetts) represent only 36 percent of the population. If we add the most conservative Democrat to that group—Senator Ben Nelson of Nebraska—that number rises to 36.3 percent.[26] Yet that minority has the power to block major legislative bills that would readily be passed by majority vote. As Paul Krugman notes:

> "America is caught between severe problems that must be addressed and a minority party determined to block action on every front. Doing nothing is not an option—not unless you want the nation to sit motionless, with an effectively paralyzed government, waiting for financial, environmental and fiscal crises to strike."[27]

9. Health care is more than just another commodity for sale on an open market.

We have allowed the health care debate to be framed as an economic issue. But it is much more—it is also a moral issue that defines the quality of our character. As far back as hundreds of years before Christ, Hippocrates in Greece was stressing the need for physicians to suppress their own self-interest and act in the best interests of their patients.[28] Dr. Edmund Pellegrino, as a physician, ethicist and moral philosopher, has reminded us for many years that:

> "Medicine is at heart a moral enterprise and those who practice it are de facto members of a moral community. We can accept or repudiate that fact, but we cannot ignore it or absolve ourselves of the moral consequences of our choice. If the care of the sick is increasingly treated as a commodity, an investment opportunity, a bureaucrat's power trip, or a political trading chip, the profession bears part of the responsibility."[29]

Few can argue today that the business ethic and profit motive have not completely taken over medicine and health care. In most parts of the system, the service ethic is long gone, surviving mainly in public safety-net programs where dedicated professionals work against the tide of their times. This book has provided many examples of exploitation of the public throughout the medical industrial complex. In his excellent book, *The Healing of America: A Global Quest for Better, Cheaper, and Fairer Health Care*, T. R. Reid has this to say:

> "When it comes to the essential task of providing health care for people, the mighty USA is a fourth-rate power... [Our country has never made a fundamental moral decision] to provide medical care for everybody who needs it."[30]

So now we find that our elected representatives in Congress, beholden as they are to corporate interests, give us a "reform" bill that will launch a new cycle of escalating profits for stakeholders, all on the backs of ordinary Americans.[31]

How we deal with this disconnect from the public interest is both a moral and political question. We are complicit with the increased hardship, suffering and premature deaths of millions of our fellow Americans if we tacitly stand by and tolerate 45,000 unnecessary deaths each year (one every 12 minutes).[32] And how should we react to the swelling ranks of the underinsured and medically bankrupt, and to the millions of our friends, neighbors and even family members delaying or going without necessary care? As Martin Luther King, Jr. observed: "Of all the forms of inequality, injustice in health care is the most shocking and most inhuman."[33]

10. Health care reform must be fundamental and comprehensive, with a simplified financing system; incrementalism has not, and will never work.

We have tried all kinds of incremental tweaks to our health care system over the last two to three decades, including virtually all of the changes incorporated in this latest "reform" bill. All have failed to arrest unaffordable inflation of health care costs or to assure access to care for all Americans. As we have discussed earlier, the entire issue of health care reform needs to be re-framed, based on a small number of principles, such as these:

- Health care, as a basic human need, should be made available to all Americans.
- Costs of health care, not just federal but also those paid by individuals and families, must be brought under control on an affordable and sustainable basis.

- Our elected representatives in government must assure universal access to health care through a public-private partnership whereby the delivery system remains private.
- Our goal should be one-tier care that maximizes the best value and outcomes of care that we can afford, both for individuals and our entire population.
- We need to replace the business ethic in health care with a service ethic as the system evolves toward a not-for-profit system.
- Bureaucracy and waste must be reduced, with at least 90 percent of the health care dollar going to direct patient care.
- Incentives among providers must be changed to discourage over-utilization of inappropriate and unnecessary services.
- Providers and manufacturers should compete on the basis of quality of care and efficacy of their products.

Our experience over the last 50-plus years tells us that a greater role of government will be required to achieve these objectives. Markets have failed to do so. The private health insurance industry has outlived its usefulness, requires government subsidies to stay alive, and no longer offers enough added value to survive. Single payer financing is the only way to assure universal access to a system reformed along the above lines. Despite the claims of opponents that such change would be too disruptive, it will be no more so than the relatively smooth transition of Medicare as it was successfully implemented in less than a year in the mid-1960s.[34]

11. We *can* afford reform, but we *cannot* afford a privately-financed market-based system.

The present market-based system has proven itself resistant to all attempts at cost containment. The 2010 "reform" bill is a bonanza for all the market stakeholders, and will just exacerbate today's cost and access problems. Along the current and inevitable trend lines, uncontrolled prices, together with over-utilization of inappropriate and unnecessary services, will bankrupt payers, whether they be public, employers, private insurers, or patients and families themselves. The "reform" package will almost certainly cost the government far more than $1 trillion over the next ten years, and many more costs will be passed along by employers and insurers to patients in skyrocketing out-of-pocket costs.

We are running record deficits at both federal and state levels. The federal government is now facing a debt approaching that of World War II, with more than $1.6 trillion in payments that were due in March 2010.[35] States cannot carry deficits forward, and face serious budget and revenue shortfalls themselves—tax revenues fell by at least 10 percent in one-half of states surveyed in the third quarter of 2009, and projections were gloomy for fiscal years 2010 and 2011.[36] Ideology aside, it should be a no-brainer to compare a health care system "reformed" by the 2010 law with the single payer option, which would:

- Guarantee universal coverage for the entire population, with full choice of physicians, other providers and hospitals without cost-sharing (all of that enabled by increasing size of the risk pool to more than 300 million and eliminating the need to build complex mechanisms to deny coverage).
- Save some $400 billion a year in administrative simplification while implementing such cost-containment measures as negotiated prices for drugs and medical devices; global budgets for hospitals and other facilities; reimbursement reform for physicians; evidence-based mechanisms for coverage and reimbursement policies; and reduction of bureaucratic barriers between patients and their physicians.
- Cost less than what employers, patients and their families are already paying for health care, allowing business to have a healthier workforce and become more competitive in a global economy, and at the same time gain more value and better outcomes of care for all Americans.
- Protect all of us from the present risk of financial ruin by one major illness or accident.

WHAT NEXT?

As we have seen, unless we shape up soon and get real, health care costs will increase the pain and suffering of a growing part of our population, further fragment us as a society, increase political backlash to the inequities of our system, and eventually bankrupt us. The stakes rise with the passing of each month and year. Despite the hype over the "reform" bill, most of its provisions will not take effect for another four or five years, and when they do they will be much less effective than we are being promised.

There is a way forward, as we will see in Chapter 11, but first we need to revisit in the next chapter the current and imminent realities that confront the next stages of health care reform.

References

1. Soros, G. The Capitalist Threat, *The Atlantic*, February, 1997.
2. Reich, R. As cited in Rothschild, M. Victory for a mediocre health care bill. *The Progressive*, March 22, 2010.
3. Reich, R. How healthcare reform makes history. *The Progressive* 15 (7): 12, April 15, 2010.
4.   Rovner, J. Republicans spurn once-favored health mandate. *NPR*, February 15, 2010.
5. MSNBC. Obama health czar directed firms in trouble: http://www.msnbc.msn.com/id/31566399/ns/health-health_care/.
6. Editorial. Puppets in Congress. *New York Times*, November 16, 2009.
7. Center for Public Integrity, as cited in Moyers, B, Winship, M. The unbearable lightness of reform. *Truthout*, March 27, 2010.
8. Giroux, HA. A society consumed by locusts: Youth in the age of moral and political plagues. *Truthout*, April 5, 2010.
9. Lerner, M. Building on the hopeful aspects of Obama's health care speech and helping him get beyond his internal contradictions. Tikkun Daily. http://www.Tikkun.org/tikkundaily/.
10. Ibid # 3.
11. Ibid # 4.
12. Johnson, A. Humana CEO keeps eye on health care reform signposts ahead. *Wall Street Journal*, November 23, 2009: B1.
13. Bodaken, B. as cited in Wolfson, B. "Vicious cycle" of care. *The Orange County Register*, March 20, 2005.
14. Hellander, I. Personal communication. April 2, 2010.
15. Geyman, JP. *Do Not Resuscitate: Why the Health Insurance Industry is Dying, and How We Must Replace It*. Monroe, ME. Common Courage Press, 2009, pp 91-121.
16. Krugman, P. California death spiral. *New York Times*, February 19, 2010: A21. Lazar, K. Short-term customers boosting health costs. *The Boston Globe*, April 4, 2010.
17. Reinhardt, UE. No such thing as 'simple' health reform. *New York Times*, January 29, 2010.
18. Randolph, L. Anthem big outlier in DMHC actions. Payers and providers. California Department of Managed Care, May 27, 2010.

19. Hellander, I. International health systems for single payer advocates. The National Health Program Reader. Leadership Training Institute. PNHP. Chicago. October 24, 2009, pp 46-7.
20. Hedges, C. *Empire of Illusion: The End of Literacy and the Triumph of Spectacle*. New York. Nation Books, 2009, p. 155.
21. Faux, J. One more bubble to go. *American Prospect* 20(10): December 2009. p.21.
22. Roosevelt, FD,Jr. as cited in Conniff, R. A deficit of leadership. *The Progressive* 74 (3): 13, 2010.
23. Gordon, C. *The Clinton Health Care Plan: Dead on Arrival*. Westfield, NJ. Open Magazine Pamphlet Series. 1995.
24. Hulse, C. A morning of Democratic glee and Republican glumness. *New York Times*, December 25, 2009: A19.
25. Krugman, P. A dangerous dysfunction. Op-Ed. *New York Times*, December 21, 2009: A29.
26. Naureckas, J. Not so fast, filibuster. Extra! December, 2009, p 5.
27. Ibid # 25.
28. Pellegrino, ED. The Hippocratic Oath and clinical ethics. *J Clin Ethics* 1 (4):290- 1, 1990.
29. Pellegrino, ED. The medical profession as a moral community. *Bull N Y Acad Med* 66 (3):222, 1990.
30. Reid, TR. *The Healing of America: A Global Quest for Better, Cheaper, and Fairer Health Care*. New York. Penguin Press, 2009.
31. Britt, R. Reform won't take bite out of health-care profits. Market Watch. *Seattle Times* on line, November 25, 2009.
32. Wilper, AP, Woolhandler, S, Lasser, K et al. Health insurance and mortality in U.S. adults. *Am J Public Health* 99, 2009.
33. King, ML, Jr. Second National Convention for the Medical Committee for Human Rights, Chicago, IL, March 25, 1966, as cited in its Volunteer Manual, available at: http://www.crmvet.org/docs/mchr.htm.accessed January 16, 2007.
34. Marmor, TF. *The Politics of Medicare*. New York. Aldine Publishing Company, 1970, p. 86.
35. Andrews, EL. Federal government faces balloon in debt payments. *New York Times*, November 23, 2009: A1.
36. Dougherty, C. States hit by drop in tax collections. *Wall Street Journal*, November 23, 2009: A4.

CHAPTER 10

New Realities: A Perfect Storm Ahead

"If one could know where we are, and whither we are tending,
we could then better judge what to do, and how to do it."

—Abraham Lincoln, 1858

As we have seen in earlier chapters, the health care system is extremely complex and difficult to restructure in terms of cost control, improved access, efficiency, quality and accountability. Much of it is for-profit and investor-owned, so that the business ethic and corporate greed tend to drive the system. Perverse incentives permeate the system so that many hospitals, other facilities and physicians earn more income—*all costs that we pay*—by providing a higher volume of services, whether necessary and appropriate or not. And the political process involved in reform attempts are even more complex, as we saw in the last chapter, whereby corporate money drowns out the voices of the electorate.

So, now that we have a health care "reform" bill that won't do the job, what can be done about it? Before dealing with that question in the next chapter, this chapter has two goals: (1) to summarize the current realities and trends still requiring fundamental health care reform; and (2) to project what we can expect to happen in the next few years as the political battle over health care reform continues.

WORSENING REALITIES AND UGLY TRENDS

In The Economy

Health care is a large part of the entire U.S. economy—more than 17 percent of the GDP, and almost one-third of the 55 percent that is the service economy. As the number of uninsured rises above 46 million and the ranks of the underinsured surge past another 30 million, more Americans are forced to rely on safety net programs, such as Medicaid and SCHIP, for which about one-quarter of the uninsured are eligible.[1]

The U.S. economy itself is in dire straits, despite the attempted optimism of those who keep telling us that the recession is almost over and that markets can fix our problems. These data points show the extent of our economic challenges:

- The projected ten-year budget deficit is $9 trillion, will be $1.5 trillion in 2010, and will remain above 3 percent of the GDP, the level that many economists believe is sustainable, for the next decade. Policymakers face a fine line—cutting the deficit too fast can depress demand and stifle our economic recovery, while cuts that are too slow can force interest rates up and also stifle the recovery.[2]
- Despite some improvements in the U.S. trade deficit, North America still has by far the widest gap between exports and imports than anywhere else in the world (13.1 vs. 18.1 percent).[3]
- The U.S. national debt is projected to nearly double to $20 trillion by 2015.[4]
- More than 40 states are *further* slashing their budgets, even after passing them earlier, due to shortfalls in tax revenues.[5] After passage of health care reform legislation, California will need an additional $3-4 billion a year.[6] As part of their budget-cutting, some states are shutting down tax credits and incentive programs intended to lure business and create jobs.[7]
- About one in four U.S. homeowners owe more on their mortgages than their properties are worth.[8]
- According to the Census Bureau, median household income (adjusted for inflation) fell 3.6 percent in 2008, the steepest annual drop in 40 years; the poverty rate of 13.2 percent (an income of $22,205 for a family of four) was highest since 1997.[9]
- Middle-class families (with annual incomes between $45,000 and $85,000) saw their median household income drop by 2.5 percent from 2000 to 2008 as their share of the cost of their family ESI health insurance increased by 81 percent.[10]
- Worries over the cost of health care are high on this list of economic concerns among Americans, as shown in Figure 10.1.[11]
- The racial gap in household net worth has soared in recent years—in 2002, median household net worth for whites was

FIGURE 10.1

Health Care Worries Are High on List

Percent saying they are "very worried" about each of the following:

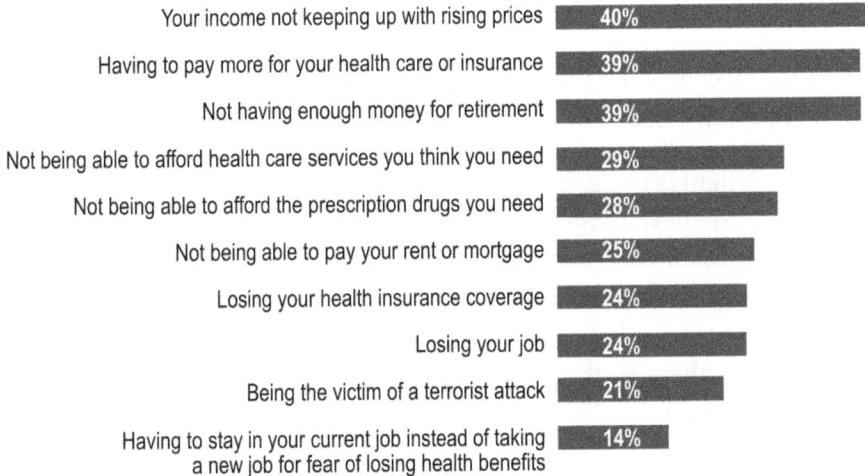

Your income not keeping up with rising prices	40%
Having to pay more for your health care or insurance	39%
Not having enough money for retirement	39%
Not being able to afford health care services you think you need	29%
Not being able to afford the prescription drugs you need	28%
Not being able to pay your rent or mortgage	25%
Losing your health insurance coverage	24%
Losing your job	24%
Being the victim of a terrorist attack	21%
Having to stay in your current job instead of taking a new job for fear of losing health benefits	14%

Source: Kaiser Health Tracking poll—March 2010 – Chartpack (#8058-C), The Henry J. Kaiser Foundation, March 2010. This information was reprinted with permission from the Henry J. Kaiser Foundation. The Kaiser Family Foundation is a non-profit private operating foundation, based in Menlo Park, California, dedicated to producing and communicating the best possible analysis and information on health issues.

about $90,000 compared to only about $8,000 for the median Latino household and $6,000 for the median black household.[12]

- The unemployment rate of close to 10 percent is actually a false low—according to the U.S. Department of Labor, the "real" num-ber (including the *underemployed* who can't find full-time work) is 17.5 percent. That's the highest since at least 1970 and most likely since the Great Depression.[13]

- Years of corporate outsourcing of jobs overseas has been a major factor in the decline of the U.S. manufacturing sector, which fell from 28 percent of our GDP in 1959 to 11.5 percent in 2008.[14]

- Small business creates two-thirds of America's new jobs, but is embroiled in a credit crunch even after the bailout of the financial industry. So future prospects are also clouded. A recent McKinsey Global Institute report found that seven of ten American workers hold jobs for which there is decreasing demand, increasing supply, or both.[15]

There is growing public awareness across the country that corporations and Wall Street have contributed in large part to our economic difficulties. Senator Bernie Sanders identifies a big problem this way:

> "It is not acceptable to me that corporate America throws millions of Americans out on the street and runs to China, pays people there 50 cents an hour, and then brings their products back to this country. We need corporate America to start investing here."[16]

Resentment is rising over Wall Street being bailed out by politicians at the expense of Main Street, and over the Obama Administration doing too little to change business as usual. This growing anger is fueled by regular press reports about the self-interest and greed of traders and investment bankers in the run-up and aftermath of the financial crisis.[17,18] Matthew Rothschild, editor of *The Progressive*, sums up the situation this way:

> "President Obama has not responded adequately to the crisis. He came in with too timid a stimulus package, one that relied on the private sector for more than 90 percent of the new jobs instead of the public sector, where the pay and benefits are higher and— not incidentally—the rate of unionization. He reacted feebly to the housing crisis. He reacted obsequiously to the banking crisis. And he's shown little appetite for the hearty re-regulation that the moment requires. Instead of fighting for economic justice, he's leaving the fundamentals of the economy just as he found them."[19]

In just a year, Wall Street had largely recovered from the crash of 2008. The stock market had rebounded strongly, the five largest remaining banks were bigger, traders and investment bankers were back to their old tricks of placing bold and risky bets with other people's money, and significant government regulation had been avoided. As already too-big-to-fail banks returned to good times, government debt loads grew larger.[20]

But the nation's real economy is still in trouble. As Robert Reich, former Secretary of Labor in the Clinton Administration and Professor of Public Policy at the University of California Berkeley, observes:

"The real locus of the problem was never the financial economy to begin with, and the bailout of Wall Street was a sideshow. The real problem was on Main Street, in the real economy. Before the crash, much of America had fallen deeply into unsustainable debt because it had no other way to maintain its standard of living. That's because for so many years almost all the gains of economic growth had been going to a relatively small number of people at the top."[21]

All of this economic turmoil is taking place in a larger context where the very concept of a global economy is being brought into question. As the well-known Canadian philosopher John Ralston Saul observed in his excellent book, *The Collapse of Globalism and the Reinvention of the World*:

"Prophets of globalization who said 'privatize, privatize, privatize' now say they were wrong, because the national rule of law is more important. Economists are angrily divided over whether to loosen or tighten controls over capital markets. Increasingly strong nation-states, like India and Brazil, are challenging the received wisdom of global economics. Pharmaceutical transnationals find themselves ducking and weaving to avoid citizen movements."[22]

In Health Care

Within the U.S. health care sector, the realities and trends are stark. Even after passage of health care "reform" legislation (Patient Protection and Affordable Care Act, PPACA), as we saw in Chapter 8, this is what we are now confronting at the start of the second decade of the new century:

- *Continued uncontrolled inflation of health care costs.* According to the annual Milliman Medical Index (MMI), the typical American family of four spent $18,074 on health care in 2010, a 7.8 percent increase over the previous year and the highest dollar increase in the last ten years. That number represents the total amount spent on actual health care for a family of four enrolled in an employer-sponsored preferred provider organization (PPO), and does *not* include the insurers' administrative expenses or profits.[23]

The CBO projects that total *federal* health care spending will grow by $965 billion over the 2010 to 2029 period.[24] Those numbers do not include the "doc fix", which will require another $200-plus billion. Nor do they include what patients and families will end up paying for health insurance and health care.

In the aftermath of the 2010 "reform" legislation, the gold rush is on! All parts of the medical industrial complex will reap a bonanza in our market-based system, accelerated by lack of price controls, perverse incentives throughout the system to do more rather than less, the persistence of high levels of inappropriate and unnecessary care, relatively lax regulation over adoption of new technologies, and the subsidizing of private insurance which will encourage insurers to further raise prices knowing Uncle Sam is helping out. As Princeton Professor Uwe Reinhardt observes: "The cost trend in health care is composed in part by utilization and in part by prices. In our market-driven system, a doctor or hospital essentially charges the maximum they can get."[25]

These three examples illustrate how these interrelated factors build on each other:

1. The pharmaceutical industry successfully avoided negotiated drug prices under health care "reform." In a November 2009 letter to the GAO, the chairmen of three House committees called out the drug industry for anticipatory price gouging in advance of the health care bill (e.g. price increases of 17 to 20 percent for such commonly used brand name drugs as Flomax, Ambien and Aricept). The latest sweepstake winner for exorbitant prices is Foltyn, Allos' new drug for pediatric leukemia, which costs $30,000 a month even though it has not yet been shown to prolong lives.[26]

2. Complex fusion procedures are becoming the latest, most invasive treatment for low back pain due to spinal stenosis. Despite a paucity of evidence for the effectiveness of this procedure, together with a high incidence of complications (5.6 percent of life-threatening complications and 13 percent rate of re-hospitalization within 30 days), the rate of this procedure

increased 15-fold from 2002 to 2007. This is the most lucrative form of treatment for that problem, both for orthopedic surgeons and for hospitals; mean hospital charges are more than $80,000 compared to $23,000 for surgical decompression alone.[27]

3. The FDA's current legal battle with ReGen Biologics gives us a good illustration of how lax regulatory controls over approval of new technologies adds to health care inflation. The company's new knee-repair device (Menaflex) was approved in December 2008 under an abbreviated review process called 510(k). The head of the FDA's medical device division approved the device over the objections of FDA scientists and managers. A subsequent investigation by the FDA found that the FDA head had "bowed to extreme pressure by members of Congress and lobbying by the company." Legal challenges have been raised over the power of the FDA to remove a previously approved product from the market, and what credence is given to the scientific review process. The outcome of litigation remains uncertain.[28]

- *Little relief in the number of uninsured for four more years*. The temporary high-risk pool will face many difficulties in implementation, and at best will not make a major dent in the number of uninsured. Many people will opt out of the individual mandate. Penalties for non-compliance won't kick in until 2014 (then at only $95, and will later max out at $695 or up to 2.5 percent of annual income in 2019). The Exchanges will not be up and running until 2014, and then will only be open to the uninsured or those working in small business without coverage. Federal subsidies for Medicaid expansion will not start until 2014. Meanwhile the number of uninsured, especially those with significant health problems, seems certain to increase as our economic problems continue.

- *Growing epidemic of underinsurance*. The addition of children to parents' policies will add more healthy people to the rolls of "insured," but usually with very limited policies without

adequate coverage if they get sick. Though we are being assured
that the new "reform" bill will remove many of the abuses
of the insurance industry, they will still have many ways to
game the system to extract maximal profits and avoid paying
for sick people. These are some of the ways: lenient medical
loss ratios of 80 to 85 percent, with new opportunities to count
other expenses as patient care (e.g. information management,
chronic disease and pay for performance initiatives); employer-
sponsored insurance plans are exempted from insurance reforms
until 2018; low requirements for their policies' actuarial value
(60 or 70 percent); and no effective controls over premium rate-
setting. Insurers will continue to target young healthier people
with barebones policies that provide little protection against
serious illness or accidents, but which are very profitable. A
2010 survey by the Kaiser Family Foundation found that the
average family deductible on the individual market was $5,149
before any coverage kicked in.[29]

- ***Continued escalation of insurance rates and unaffordability of
  coverage.*** We have known for years that rising health care costs
  are diverting wage increases for many millions of Americans.
  Figure 10.2 shows us the impacts of household health care
  spending compared to average income over the years between
  1980 and 2007.[30] This trend will continue in coming years.
  Despite the absence of significant inflation and recessionary
  conditions, health insurers in 2010 are increasing their premium
  costs by 10 to 13 percent, depending on type of plan.[31] For
  workers covered by employer-sponsored insurance, their share
  of premiums increased by 10 percent in 2010.[32] The CBO has
  projected that the family insurance premium in the ESI market
  in 2016 will cost more than $20,000, *not* including deductibles
  and other out-of-pocket costs.[33] People on private Medicare
  Advantage plans will see their benefits cut and premiums rise,
  since almost one-third of proposed Medicare cuts will phase
  down overpayments to these programs. And AHIP has already
  warned that weakening of the individual mandate will require
  insurers to continue to increase their premiums in future years to
  cover their "cost burden."

  When subsidized coverage begins in 2014, we can anticipate

FIGURE 10.2

Impact of Household Health Care Spending on Income, 1980 - 2007

Thousands of Dollars*

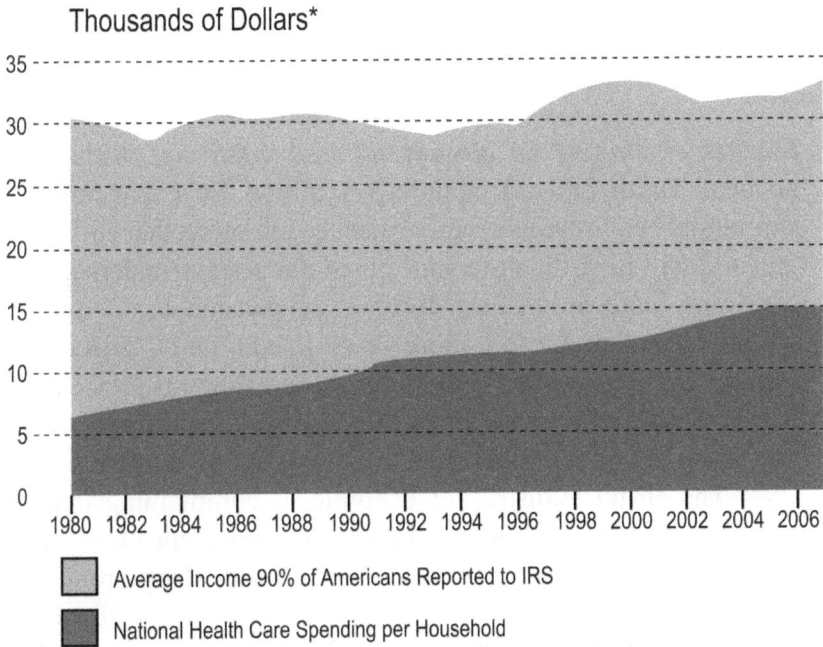

Average Income 90% of Americans Reported to IRS

National Health Care Spending per Household

* Adjusted for inflation to 2008 dollars

Source: Reprinted with permission from Johnson, DC. By the numbers. *The Nation* 289 (8): 5, September 21, 2009.

some decrease in the number of people filing for bankruptcy due to health care costs. But among the subset of those who file for bankruptcy who have insurance, that number will likely remain high, or even increase.

- *Excessive cost-cutting in the service of a business model to increase profits is hazardous to patients.* The Senate Finance Committee conducted an investigation in 2010 into patient deaths and allegations of sub-standard treatment at long-term care hospitals. Select Medical Corporation is a for-profit corporation that runs 89 long-term care hospitals in the U.S., more than any other company. Medicare pays about $5 billion a year on these hospitals, comprising about 60 percent of their total revenue. The investigation called into question the company's staffing, patient monitoring and emergency care. In one incident, a dying patient's cardiac alarm sounded for 77 minutes before nurses responded. Former employees have said that the facilities are understaffed and depend on temporary nurses. Select Medical has reported that it raised its profit margin by 19 percent in 2009.[34]

- ***Further erosion of an already tattered safety net***. Although the final health bill did include $11 billion for expansion of community health centers, a much needed initiative, that will take time and will be difficult to staff given our serious undersupply of primary care providers. Moreover, expansion of Medicaid will not take place for four more years. In addition, COBRA, as a temporary (18 months) backup for those losing insurance and their jobs, will still not be affordable for many Americans, even with extended government subsidies covering 65 percent of its costs. The HMO industry, for example, is complaining that it loses 200 percent of premium income on those enrollees, and will likely pass these losses on to patients with sharp premium increases.[35]

Many states are already in severe financial distress, and are appealing to the federal government for additional help. In response to this crisis, more than one-half of states are delaying full payment into their pension plans for state employees, thereby "kicking the can" down the road.[36] In Louisiana, officials are saying that reduced federal funds to hospitals that treat the uninsured can be a death knell for its state-run charity hospital system. In California, Kim Belshe, secretary of the Department of Health and Human Services agency (DHHS), warns: "The federal government has to account for states' inability to sustain our current programs, much less expand."[37]

- ***Impending collapse of our primary care infrastructure even as the nation looks to double Medicaid enrollment over the next eight years.*** We have seen earlier how most of the physician workforce has gravitated over many years to higher-paying non-primary care specialties with more comfortable lifestyles and are mightily encouraged in that direction by onerous school loans required to pay for medical school. It is estimated that the U.S. will have a shortage of 35,000 to 44,000 primary care practitioners for adults by 2025.[38] Primary care physicians today are overwhelmed with patients and bureaucratic paperwork, leading to increasing stress and, for many, early retirement. Many patients have a difficult time finding a primary care physician to take care of them, forcing them to confront a confusing multi-specialty system without enough continuity of care. A recent survey by the Commonwealth Fund of primary care physicians in 11 countries provides a useful snapshot of the current situation with interesting cross-national comparisons. U.S. primary care physicians are much less available to their patients after hours than their counterparts in other countries and are far more burdened with administrative tasks. Their patients have more difficulty in paying for medical care. Timely access to specialists is the main advantage for U.S. patients, but the other side of that coin is the comparative lack of comprehensive primary care, as well as the attendant costs and the discontinuity of specialty care.[39]

- ***Increasing mortality and morbidity with decreasing health status.*** We already know that some 45,000 Americans die each year as a consequence of being uninsured.[40] Two million patients with cancer are foregoing medical services each year due to unaffordable costs.[41] A recent study even found that more than 2,200 uninsured U.S. military veterans under the age of 65 died because of decreased access to care.[42] Moreover, we know that uninsured people with such chronic diseases such as hypertension and diabetes are at much higher risk of major complications as a result of reduced access to medical care.[43] In view of the four-year delay in implementing many of the "reforms" in the new health care bill, these numbers are not likely to turn around and may even get worse. Another useful benchmark is self-perceived health status as a subjective measure of personal health. This too has been in decline for many years. The proportion of U.S. adults under age 65 reporting excellent or very good health dropped from 64 to 56 percent between 1993 and 2007, despite per capita health care spending that more than doubled over that period.[44]

• *Poor cross-national comparisons of system performance.* With its multi-payer, profit-oriented market-based system, the U.S. spends far more per-capita on health care than any other country in the world, double what many advanced countries pay while achieving better outcomes than we do. A big part of this problem is the high prices that are charged throughout our system. Actually, despite our enormous spending on health care, the U.S. has fewer health care resources per capita than the international average for 30 countries in the Organization for Economic Cooperation and Development (OECD)—fewer total numbers of physicians and nurses, fewer physician visits, fewer hospital beds and shorter hospital stays per capita.[45] The U.S. does not fare well in other cross-national comparisons. These examples show how little value we get from our enormously expensive, profit-driven system compared with other industrialized countries:

1. The U.S. ranks last among 19 industrialized countries in "amenable mortality rates", deaths that could have been prevented by timely and effective health care. That dry statistic translates to about 101,000 excessive deaths per year in this country.[46]

2. The U.S. also ranks last among 23 industrialized nations on infant mortality, with rates more than double those of Iceland, Japan and France.[47]

3. Lower-income people in the U.S. receive worse care than their higher-income counterparts on 21 of 30 primary care quality measures, four to five times higher rates of disparity compared to Canada and Australia.[48]

4. Patients in this country are more likely than those in seven other countries to say that they have experienced medical errors or went without needed care because of costs. More than one-third of Americans believe that our health care system needs to be "rebuilt completely," compared to 15 percent in the U.K. and 12 percent in Canada.[49]

5. In an international survey of patient views on the care they

receive, U.S. patients scored their care the worst on four of the six Institute of Medicine quality measures: patient safety, patient-centeredness, efficiency, and equity.[50]

In sum, the major problems requiring reform in the first place— soaring costs of insurance and health care, growing unaffordability, inadequate access and variable quality of care—will be largely unchanged by the "reform" legislation. The adverse impacts on patients and families will continue, and for many get worse. What does all this bode for the public reaction and the political process?

AN ONGOING POLITICAL BATTLE OVER HEALTH CARE

As the new health care law begins to take effect, the political wars go on without interruption, both between and among the corporate stakeholders and between the political parties as they try to gain advantage during the 2010 election cycle.

Battles within the Medical-Industrial Complex

It will take months for some of the important details to be clarified, so lobbyists for each industry will keep up the pressure to seek industry-friendly treatment. More than 40 provisions of PPACA require or permit government agencies to issue rules. The Secretary for Health and Human Services, for example, is responsible for defining the breadth of coverage in an "essential benefits package," as well as determining the rules by which insurers will calculate how much they spend on direct medical care, their MLRs. Insurers are already pressing for loose definitions of "direct medical care," hoping to include spending on health information technology, nurse hot lines, care review by physicians and hospitals, quality improvement activities and anti-fraud efforts. All would add to their financial bottom lines if counted as direct medical care.[51]

Meanwhile, stakeholders are fighting among themselves to maximize their profits. Insurers are taking a more aggressive stance against hospitals in their contract agreements. For example, a unit of WellPoint recently dropped the Stellaris Health Network, a four-hospital chain in Westchester, New York from its network after Stellaris asked for a 15 percent increase in reimbursement payments. Arthur Nizza, Stellaris president and CEO, said: "Our non-profit community hospitals can no longer subsidize the record profits of a health insurance conglomerate."[52] Insurers are also suing state regulators over what they consider restrictions on premium rate decisions, including Massachusetts, Maine and Pennsylvania.[53-55] Meanwhile, AHIP is embarking on a new 50-state effort to *Enroll America,* seeking the most rigorous implementation of the individual mandate with the most generous subsidies by government.[56]

As insurers up the ante in their dealings with hospitals and physicians, they get stronger pushback from those groups. The AMA argues that the insurance industry has become much too consolidated, and rails against its "take it or leave it" approach to contracts. In an updated report based on 2009 data, the AMA found that 99 percent of 313 metropolitan areas were "highly concentrated" under guidelines used by the U.S. Department of Justice and the Federal Trade Commission; one insurer holds more that 70 percent of the market in 24 of 43 states measured.[57]

More physicians are leaving private practice every year as the administrative burdens multiply, seeking out salaried jobs with hospitals and health systems with more bargaining clout. Less than one-half of medical practices in this country are physician-owned, a big drop from previous years.[58]

But the tensions between physicians and hospitals are ratcheting up all the time. One recent example is the termination of the contracts of two primary care internists by the Chief Financial Officer of the St. John Medical Center in Westlake, Ohio for "not being sufficiently productive" (i.e. not ordering enough tests or admitting enough patients to the hospital). The two board-certified internists cared for about 2,500 patients, in some cases over more than 20 years. They had excellent records with the hospital, never had an unfavorable review, and had high patient satisfaction and retention rates. The medical staff had been previously requested to "admit just one more Medicare patient a month" to the hospital to help the hospital's finances. Some physicians had questioned the moral justification and legal propriety of that request. A firestorm of protest erupted over this termination, and the Mobilize Ohio Movement, a single payer activist organization, staged a rally to demand the reinstatement of the two physicians.[59]

Employers are taking a hard look at the new health care bill, and already are concerned about adverse impacts. For example, large companies have been benefiting from a little-known provision in the 2003 Medicare prescription drug bill (MMA) that provides them with a $28 subsidy for every $100 they spend on retiree drug coverage. Since the subsidy was tax-free, they received a double-tax break in deducting the full $100 as a business expense. While the new health care legislation retains the subsidy, companies can no longer deduct it as their own business expense.[60] Although small businesses welcome their tax credits, many worry that what they may save in costs in the short term may subject them to higher taxes in the longer term. As Molly Brogan, vice president of public affairs for the National Small Business Association, says: "The health care law certainly addresses a lot of the access side of the equation, but it doesn't address costs."[61]

Portents for the 2010 Elections

In view of the sharp split in public opinion towards health care reform legislation and the complete polarization between political parties, both sides are making health care a major issue in the 2010 election cycle.

Republicans seek to portray the new law as lacking in popular support, a long-term deficit buster, and a gross overreach of government power. While Republicans are correct in recognizing the lack of significant cost containment in the new bill, their alternate plan has no chance of reforming our system. Their approach is to trust the market, provide vouchers, cut Medicare funds, pass more costs and responsibility on to patients, and reduce the role of government in health care.[62] They wait in the wings for PPACA to fail and then call for increased privatization as the solution, ignoring the inconvenient fact that PPACA is really a Republican plan mirrored after the supposed "Massachusetts Miracle" enacted by Republican Governor Mitt Romney in 2006.

Democrats are trying to better explain the contents of the complex legislation and tout the ways in which it will help many millions of Americans.[63] That task is difficult in view of the small number of "early deliverables" of PPACA and the continued soaring costs and prices of health care.

As *New York Times* columnist Charles Blow predicted in mid-November 2009 about the 2010 elections:

"The party that wins the White House generally loses Congressional seats in the midterm, but this Democrat-controlled government has particular issues. Its agenda has been hamstrung by a perfect storm of politics: the Republicans' surprisingly effective obstructionist strategy, a Democratic caucus riddled with conservative sympathizers and a president encircled by crises and crippled by caution."[64]

With the New Year, there was wide consensus that the midterm elections would be turbulent and hard-fought. While Democrats fear the loss of some seats in Congress, they are determined to keep their majority in the House, where Republicans would have to gain 41 seats to gain control.[65] But with growing numbers of legislators in both parties deciding to retire, the midterm elections are expected to be closer than previously thought. Democratic senators face serious challenges in such swing states as Pennsylvania, Illinois, Arkansas, Colorado and Nevada, while retirements are putting other states in play, such as North Dakota and Indiana.[66]

There was no lull in the political wars when the health care legislation was signed into law. Within minutes, attorneys general from 13 states filed a lawsuit in Pensacola against the federal government, alleging that the individual mandate is unconstitutional.[67] Corporate stakeholders announced their campaigns to influence the November elections over health care issues—the Chamber of Commerce with a $50 million effort targeting pivotal House and Senate races; AHIP pressing for industry-friendly fine print in the regulations yet to be written; the AMA opposing cuts in Medicare payments; and the AFL-CIO with a $53 million campaign.[68] Death threats were reported against some legislators who had voted both for and against the new law. And fresh battles erupted in many states over abortion coverage, with lawmakers in six states promoting legislation that would block abortion coverage in some health plans.[69]

Health care reform remains a polarizing issue across the political spectrum. A *USA Today*/Gallup poll a week after the law was signed found that 58 percent of respondents believed the legislation would not control health care costs. Beyond that, both sides could claim popular support for their views—for example, 65 percent thought there would be too much expansion of the government in health care, while 52 percent felt there should have been a public option and 51 percent believed that the bill doesn't go far enough in regulating the health care industries.[70] About the same time, a CBS News poll found that President Obama's approval rating on health care fell to a personal low—just 34 percent. As David Herszenhorn of the *New York Times* observed:

> "Health care is an issue that many Americans feel strongly about, but it also became a touchstone, a proxy for larger disagreements and deeper divisions in an increasingly fractured society."[71]

Little more than six months before the midterm elections, their outcome appears both unpredictable and probably closer than previously thought. Pollster Neil Newhouse noted that when presidents had approval ratings of less than 50 percent, their parties lost an average of 41 House seats in midterm elections—an April 2010 Gallup Poll put Obama at 45 percent. In addition, of the last nine presidents before Obama, none saw their approval ratings go up between January and October of their first midterm year. So if history were to be any kind of guide, a major shift in governance would not be out of the question.[72]

Projections for 2020 Without Fundamental Reform

One does not need to be a rocket scientist to accurately predict the future of our health care system. Its adverse trends are so well entrenched and resistant to past incremental reform efforts that, in the absence of real reform, we can project them to their inevitable outcomes with confidence.

In 2000, the Institute of the Future published a book, *Health and Health Care 2010: The Forecast, the Challenges*. It described three possible scenarios for 2010. Its worst scenario, stormy weather, is what actually has come about:

- spending growth 2.5 percent above nominal GDP
- managed care fails to control costs or improve quality
- M.D./consumer backlash
- gaming and adverse selection in private Medicare plans
- hospital oligopolies sustain high prices
- large employers pay up, small ones drop insurance benefits
- new medical technologies are costly and in high demand
- HIT systems costly and ineffective
- no social consensus of limiting end-of-life spending

- safety net in tatters

All of these projections were spot-on; they surround us today as the worst of the three scenarios.[73]

TABLE 10.1

Alternative Scenarios For 2020

	Multi-Payer (2010 Health Care "Reform")	Single Payer (H.R. 676)
Universal coverage?	No. 23 million uninsured, many millions underinsured.	Yes. Automatic for all Americans.
Cost containment?	No. Out of control, with no remedy in sight.	Yes. Made possible by $400 billion a year in administrative savings, bulk purchasing, and negotiated fees and budgets in a not-for-profit system.
Affordability?	No. Severe rationing by ability to pay; high cost-sharing; increased medical bankruptcies.	Yes. No cost-sharing; patients and employers pay less than they do now.
Comprehensive Benefits?	No. Severe tiering by actuarial value of coverage.	Yes. For all necessary and effective care.
Free Choice of Doctor and Hospital?	No. Many restrictions in volatile health plans.	Yes. Anywhere in the country.
Quality of Care?	Highly variable; 23,000 additional deaths a year; increased public dissatisfaction.	Improved, through universal access and reduction of inappropriate and unnecessary care.
Bureaucracy?	Greatly increased.	Greatly reduced.
Equity?	No. Increased disparities.	Yes. Builds social solidarity.
Sustainability?	No. Widespread system collapse.	Yes. Through simplified administration in more accountable system.

In earlier chapters we have seen how the 2009-2010 reform effort was hijacked by corporate interests and their allies in their successful effort to retain the status quo of a largely deregulated marketplace while keeping a failing profit-driven private health insurance industry alive through increased government subsidies. So we can safely predict what will happen by 2020 unless real reform is undertaken, enabled by publicly financed Medicare for All, harnessed to the strengths of our private delivery system. Table 10.1 summarizes what we can expect for each scenario.

With a clearer understanding of the new realities and challenges, it is now time to move on to Part III, where we will sketch out a road map to lasting reform of our very sick system.

References

1. Adamy, J. Government becoming insurer for more people. *Wall Street Journal*, September 11, 2009: A3.
2. McKinnon, JD. Big budget deficits demand number crunching, and more. *Wall Street Journal*, December 29, 2009: A14.
3. Kalwarski, T. Penny-pinching Americans downsize the trade deficit. *BusinessWeek*, November 16, 2009: 025.
4. United States public debt. 2010 Budget. As cited in Wikopedia, accessed January 1, 2010.
5. Merrick, A. States scramble to close new budget gaps. *Wall Street Journal*, December 18, 2009: A6.
6. Woo, S. California pushes for federal help. *Wall Street Journal*, December 31, 2009: A4.
7. Dougherty, C. States cut tax incentives for new business. *Wall Street Journal*, May 10, 2010: A8.
8. Simon, R, Hagerty, JR. 1 in 4 borrowers under water. *Wall Street Journal*, November 24, 2009: A1.
9. Dougherty, C. Recession takes toll on living standards. *Wall Street Journal*, September 11, 2009: A3.
10. *USA Today* on line. Survey shows how middle class hit by health-insurance crisis. March 17, 2010.
11. Kaiser Family Foundation. Tracking Poll, March 2010)
12. Hamilton, D, Darity, W., Jr. Race, wealth, and intergenerational poverty. *The American Prospect* 20 (7): A10, September, 2009.
13. Leonhardt, D. Jobless rate hits 10.2 %, with more underemployed. *New York Times*, November 7, 2009: A1.
14. McCormick, R. The plight of American manufacturing. *The American Prospect* 20 (1): January-February, 2009: A3.

15. Foroohar, R. Joblessness is here to stay. *Newsweek,* December 21, 2009: 53.
16. Sanders, B. These people have no shame. *The Progressive* 73 (12): 41, December 2009/January 2010.
17. Story, L. Executives kept wealth as firms failed, study says. *New York Times,* November 23, 2009: B3.
18. Enrich, D, Craig, S. Shh! Wall Street is spending again. *Wall Street Journal,* November 30, 2009: C1.
19. Rothschild, M. Beyond the greed economy. *The Progressive* 73 (12): 8, December 2009/January 2010.
20. Whitehouse, M. Economists see crisis response as risky. *Wall Street Journal,* January 6, 2009: A2.
21. Reich, R. 2009: The year Wall Street bounced back and Main Street got shafted. Truthout, December 27, 2009.
22. Saul, JR. *The Collapse of Globalism and the Reinvention of the World.* New York. The Overlook Press, 2005, pp. 3-4, 2005.
23. Milliman, Inc. 2010 Milliman Medical Index, May 12, 2010.
24. CBO. The health care law. Questioning the cost of the health care overhaul. *New York Times,* April 3, 2010: A11.
25. Reinhardt, UW. As cited in Boulton, G. Insurers alone can't be blamed for rates, economists say. *Milwaukee Journal Sentinel* on line. March 13, 2010.
26. Pollack, A. A fortune to fight cancer. *New York Times,* December 5, 2009: B1.
27. Deyo, RA, Mirza, SK, Martin, BI, Kreuter, W, Goodman, DC et al. Trends, major medical complications, and charges associated with surgery for lumbar spinal stenosis in older adults. *JAMA* 303 (13): 1259-65, 2010.
28. Mundy, A. FDA wrestles with undoing decision. *Wall Street Journal,* March 22, 2010: B1.
29. Kaiser Family Foundation. Recent premium increases imposed by insurers averaged 20 % for people who buy their own health insurance. June 21, 2010.
30. Johnson, DC. By the numbers. *The Nation* 289 (8): 5, September 21, 2009.
31. Moeller, P. Double-digit medical expense trend to continue. *U.S.News & World Report,* September 3, 2009.
32. Arnst, C. Health costs: steeper still. *BusinessWeek,* October 19, 2009.
33. Congressional Budget Office. *An Analysis of Health Insurance Premiums Under the Patient Protection and Affordable Care Act.* November 30, 2009.
34. Berenson, A. Senate panel to investigate deaths at long-term care facilities. *New York Times,* March 9, 2010: B1.
35. Whelan, D. COBRA ache. A pain in the wallet. *Forbes,* November 2, 2009: 32.
36. Chon, G. States skip pension payments, delay day of reckoning. *Wall Street Journal,* April 9, 2010: A5.
37. Luo, M. Some states find burdens in health law. *New York Times,* March 27, 2010: A1.
38. Colwill, JM, Cultice, JM, Kruse, RL. Will generalist physician supply meet demands of an increasing and aging population? *Health Aff (Millwood)* 27: w232- 41, 2008.
39. Schoen, C, Osborn, R, Doty, MM, Squires, D, Peugh, J et al. A survey of

primary care physicians in eleven countries, 2009: Perspectives on care, costs, and experiences. *Health Affairs Web Exclusive*, W1171-83, 2009.

40. Wilper, AP, Woolhandler, S, Lasser, K, McCormick, D, Bor, DH et al. Health insurance and mortality in U.S. adults. *American Journal of Public Health*, September 17, 2009.

41. Weaver, KE, Roland, JH, Bellizzi, KM, Ariz, NM. Foregoing medical care because of cost: Assessing disparities in healthcare access among cancer survivors living in the United States. *Cancer* online, June 14, 2010

42. Woolhandler, S, Himmelstein, DU. Over 2,200 veterans died in 2008 due to lack of health insurance. Press release. Chicago, Ill. Physicians for a National Health Program, November 10, 2009.

43. Wilper, AP, Woolhandler, S, Lasser, K, McCormick, D, Bor, DH et al. Hypertension, diabetes, and elevated cholesterol among insured and uninsured U.S. adults. *Health Affairs*, October 20, 2009.

44. Rabin, D, Petterson, SM, Bazemore, AW, Teevan, B, Phillips, RL et al. Decreasing self-perceived health status despite rising health expenditures. *American Family Physician* 80 (5): 427, 2009.

45. Anderson, GF, Frogner, BK, Reinhardt, UE. Health spending in OECD countries in 2004: An update. *Health Affairs* 26 (5): 1481-9, 2007.

46. Nolte, E, McKee, CM. U.S. has most preventable deaths among 19 nations. *Health Affairs* 27 (1): 58-71, 2008.

47. Schoen, C, Davis, K, How, SKH, Schoenbaum, SC. U.S. health system performance: A national scorecard. *Health Affairs Web Exclusive*, W457-475, 2006.

48. Huynh, P et al. The U.S. health care divide. Commonwealth Fund, April, 2006.

49. Mahon, M. International Survey: U.S. adults most likely to report medical errors and skip needed care due to costs. One third of U.S. adults call for completely rebuilding the health care system. New York. Commonwealth Fund, November 1, 2007.

50. Davis, K et al. Mirror, mirror on the wall. Commonwealth Fund, April, 2006.

51. Pear, R. Health insurance companies try to shape rules. *New York Times*, May 16, 2010: A17.

52. Johnson, A, Sataline, S. WellPoint unit drops Stellaris from network. *Wall Street Journal*, April 2, 2010.

53. Weisman, R. Insurers call halt, get state warning. *The Boston Globe* on line, April 7, 2010.

54. Mathews, AW, Johnson, A. Insurer fights Maine regulator on premiums. *Wall Street Journal*, April 2, 2010: B1.

55. Berry, E. Highmark sues to block state review of Blues competition. *American Medical News,* April 5, 2010.

56. Scherer, M. Once opponents, insurers back effort to make health reform succeed. *Time* Search Time.com, March 24, 2010.

57. Berry, E. Health plans extend their market dominance. *American Medical News*, March 8, 2010.

58. Harris, G. More doctors giving up private clinics. *New York Times*, March 26, 2010.

59. Smith, D. Press release. Patients, physicians and health care activists to protest St. John Medical Center's plans to eliminate primary care practices. Mobilize Ohio Movement. April 29, 2010. Available at www.mobilizeohio.org.

60. Editorial. We call that double-dipping. *New York Times*, April 6, 2010: A22.

61. Khan, H. Will new health care law really help small business? *ABC News* on line, April 2, 2010.

62. Cohn, J. Yes, let's talk about those Republican ideas. *Kaiser Health News*, February 8, 2010.

63. Bendavid, N. Both parties to highlight bill in bid to win over 2010 voters. *Wall Street Journal*, December 26-27, 2009: A4.

64. Blow, C. The passion of the right. *New York Times*, November 14, 2009:A21.

65. Wallsten, P. Democrats' blues grow deeper in new poll. *Wall Street Journal*, December 17, 2009: A8.

66. Bendavid, N. Elections' stakes: control of Senate. *Wall Street Journal*, February 17, 2010: A6.

67. Leopold. J. Obama signs health care overhaul into law. *Truthout*, March 23, 2010.

68. Adamy, J. Business bids to shape health changes. *Wall Street Journal*, March 31, 2020: A4.

69. Mathews, AW. Health overhaul reignites abortion fight at state level. *Wall Street Journal*, April 8, 2010: A6.

70. Page, S. Health care law too costly, most say. *USA TODAY*, March 30, 2010, 1A.

71. Herszenhorn, DM. As overhaul passes, the vitriol lives on. *New York Times*, March 29, 2010: A13)

72. Harwood, J. Conflicting signs for midterm elections. *New York Times*, April 12, 2010: A16.

73. Institute for the Future. *Health and Health Care 2010: The Forecast, the Challenges*. San Francisco. Jossey-Bass Publishers, 2000: 123-137 and Appendix.

PART III

A Road Map to Reform
Based on Single Payer Financing

PART III

CHAPTER 11

Déjà Vu All Over Again:
A Century Of Health Care Reform
Attempts in America

"The evidence is conclusive that our people do not yet receive all the benefits they could from modern medicine. For the rich and near-rich there is no real problem since they can command the very best science has to offer... Among the majority of the population, however, there are great islands of untreated or partially treated cases... Although it is a principle of far-reaching and, perhaps, of revolutionary significance, I think there are few who would deny that our ultimate objective should be to make these benefits available in full measure to all of the people."

— Ray Lyman Wilbur, M.D., first Dean of the Stanford Medical School,
President of Stanford University, 1916 to 1943, Chairman of the Committee
on the Costs of Medical Care (CCMC) during the Great Depression.[1]

The above conclusion was reached by Dr. Wilbur in 1932 in the interim report of the CCMC entitled *The Economics of Public Health and Medical Care*. It is too bad that his wisdom has been ignored by policy makers and politicians for almost 80 years. It appears that we have to discover old truths for ourselves the old fashioned way—by further trial and especially error. As Aaron Wildavsky, Professor of Political Science and founding dean of the Graduate School of Public Policy at the University of California Berkeley reminds us:

"If history is abolished, nothing is settled. Old quarrels become new conflicts... Doing without history is a little like abolishing memory—momentarily convenient, perhaps—but ultimately embarrassing."[2]

If we had learned anything from history before embarking on this latest attempt to reform health care in this country, we might have avoided some of the pitfalls that brought down previous attempts. So it is not just useful, but essential, that we now look to our history before thinking about how to be more successful next time.

This chapter undertakes three goals: (1) to briefly review five major attempts since 1912 to enact some form of national health insurance; (2) to describe changing political dynamics in terms of stakeholders and stake challengers; and (3) to show how this latest 2009-10 attempt fits historical patterns and offers lessons that should guide future reform efforts.

FIVE MAJOR ATTEMPTS TO ENACT NATIONAL HEALTH INSURANCE

First Attempt: 1912-1917

In 1912, President Theodore Roosevelt campaigned on the Progressive Party ticket for national health insurance (NHI), together with women's suffrage, safe conditions for industrial workers and other social issues.[3] This would have been consistent with a trend over the previous 30 years in many European countries to establish one form or another of social health insurance.[4] Although Teddy Roosevelt lost the election to Woodrow Wilson, progressives continued to push for NHI over the next few years. Several states, including Massachusetts, New York and California, introduced health insurance bills during those years, and Congress held hearings in 1916 on a federal plan to provide disability and sickness benefits.[5]

Some reform groups, including a strong American Association for Labor Legislation (AALL), advocated energetically for NHI. But as the public debate proceeded, some of the initial proponents for NHI developed conflicting positions. Organized labor, for example, later sided more with business. Then with a sudden shift of the country's priorities with our entry into World War I, the proposal was defeated in 1917 by a powerful alliance between business and organized medicine. In his later analysis of this defeat, Paul Starr concluded that contributing factors included American attitudes of individualism and self-reliance as well as weaker presidential power compared to heads of state in such countries as England and Germany.[6]

Second Attempt: 1932-1938

The 1920s saw a growing concern across the country about the rising costs of health care. As a result, an independent commission was established with private funding, the Committee on the Costs of Medical Care (CCMC), including economists, physicians and public health professionals. For a growing number of families during those Great Depression years, average family costs of care ($250 a year) consumed one-third or more of their annual income. Chaired by Dr. Ray Lyman Wilbur, the Commission issued an influential interim report in 1932, *The Economics of Public Health and Medical Care,* calling for "a new approach to health insurance because the costs of medical care now involve larger sums of money and affect more people than does wage-loss due to sickness."[7]

As the CCMC led the charge for NHI, the American Medical Association (AMA) quickly denounced it as socialism. President Franklin D. Roosevelt had already successfully taken on the special interests in enacting the Glass-Steagall Act, divesting Wall Street investment houses of banking functions, and by establishing the Tennessee Valley Authority to provide cheap electric power in the South. He was reluctant, however, to take on the AMA over NHI. The AMA was a much more consolidated and powerful group than it is today, so the New Deal went ahead with Social Security without NHI. Of special interest today, however, is that FDR was fully prepared to fight for legislation without a bipartisan approach. In her classic biography, *FDR,* Jean Edward Smith, Professor of Political Science at Marshall University, describes how FDR relished the hatred of the special interests, whom he called "economic royalists," and waged class warfare without apology as long as he knew he had a majority of the public on his side.[8]

Imagine how different a place we would be in today had President Obama adopted FDR's leadership style in welcoming "hatred of the special interests" and built his campaign for health care reform on the lessons of history with a willingness to take on the opponents of reform.

Third Attempt: 1945-1950

While postponing action on NHI during the 1930s, FDR did not abandon the idea. He put it back on the legislative agenda in his 1944 State of the Union message, asking Congress for an "economic bill of rights" to include a plan for adequate medical care.[9] After FDR died in April 1945, President Harry Truman proposed a compulsory plan for comprehensive NHI, together with increased hospital construction and doubling the numbers of physicians and nurses nationwide.[10] NHI was to be administered through the Social Security program, and its provisions were incorporated into the Wagner-Murray-Dingell bill in Congress.[11]

Battle lines over the latest proposal for NHI were quickly drawn, pitting the AMA and American Hospital Association (AHA) against progressives and the Committee on the Nation's Health, an ad hoc group of liberals and union leaders.[12] While President Truman attempted to reassure opponents that the program would not be socialized medicine and that "people would get medical and hospital services just as they do now," opponents demonized the bill as socialism. The AMA went so far as to claim that NHI would "turn physicians into slaves," proposing instead an expansion of voluntary health insurance and indigent care services.[13,14]

The AMA and AHA led a well-funded campaign against the bill, joining with large corporations, the American Bar Association, the Chamber of Commerce, and community organizations in the effort.[15] Most of the country's press was sympathetic to the opposition. Predictably, as the acrimonious debate wore on, public attitudes toward NHI, while favorable among 58 percent of the public in 1945, eroded in later surveys as a majority of people turned to favor *voluntary* health insurance.[16] The third attempt to enact NHI lost public and legislative support as the nation entered the Korean War.

Although no further attempts were made during the 1950s and 1960s to push for NHI, a number of important advances were made legislatively toward the goals of health care reform, including these significant events:

- 1950: Amendments to the Social Security Act permitting federal "vendor payments" to the states as matching funds for medical care of welfare recipients, the forerunner of Medicaid.[17,18]
- 1954: The Internal Revenue Act exempts employee benefits, such as health insurance and pensions, from income taxes.[19]
- 1962: President John F. Kennedy proposes a national health insurance plan for Social Security recipients; this was killed in Congress by strong lobbying from the medical industry.[20]
- 1965: Following the Democrats' sweep of Congress in the 1964 elections, and the increasing influence of labor unions and the civil rights movement, Medicare and Medicaid were enacted as

part of President Lyndon B. Johnson's Great Society programs to provide health care coverage to people 65 years of age and older as well as the poor.[21]

- 1968: U.S. Supreme Court recognized "an acknowledged right to health derived from a constitutionally guaranteed right to life and happiness;" conservatives argued that the right to health care is a "qualified right granted patients but modified by the available resources within the health care system and the rights of physicians to control the practice of their profession."[22,23]

Fourth Attempt: 1971-1974

Health insurance returned to the national stage in 1971 when President Richard M. Nixon proposed an employer mandate, a "play or pay" plan requiring employers to either provide a minimal level of health insurance coverage to their employees or pay a tax that would finance their coverage from an insurance pool that would also cover the unemployed. That plan would have also placed a ceiling on out-of-pocket health care expenses and eliminated exclusions based on pre-existing conditions. In addition, it called for the widespread adoption of health maintenance organizations (HMOs) with the goal to cover 90 percent of the population by 1980. An accompanying "Family Health Insurance Program" would have subsidized basic coverage for low-income families, thereby replacing Medicaid. Senator Edward M. Kennedy counter-proposed the "Health Security Act," a single payer public financing system for universal coverage of all Americans.[24,25] True to form, the AMA put forward its own Medicredit proposal, which would have provided tax credits to help people buy their own private insurance.[26]

These proposals generated furious debate. Liberals considered the Nixon proposal a windfall for the private insurance industry that fell short of universal coverage by 20 to 40 million people, while conservatives held out for a much more limited role of government. A compromise proposal was forged between Kennedy and Representative Wilbur Mills (D-AR), the powerful Chairman of the House Ways and Means Committee, that would have required co-payments of 25 percent and put an annual cap of $1,000 on health care payments by individuals or families.[27]

While the Kerr-Mills bill came quite close to passage, other events soon claimed the country's attention, especially the Vietnam War, Watergate, and Mills' personal scandal over Fannie Fox. As Paul Starr later noted: "If the name on the plan had not been Nixon and had the time not been the year of Watergate, the United States might have had national health insurance in 1974."[28]

Instead, the Health Maintenance Organization Act was finally passed in December 1973, setting aside $375 million for a five-year demonstration project to test the feasibility of HMOs. This was followed the next year by the Employee Retirement Income Security Act (ERISA), which exempted large corporations' self-insured health plans from state regulations.[29]

Fifth Attempt: 1993-1994

Although Jimmy Carter campaigned for NHI during the 1976 presidential elections, health care soon lost its priority on the national agenda as the country was forced to deal with a recession and inflation. Carter's loss to Ronald Reagan in 1980 ushered in a new time of conservative dominance, accompanied by a resurgence of corporatization of market-based health care with little regulation. Reagan's philosophy had been clearly enunciated 20 years earlier: "Medicare is not just the first step toward a total government takeover of medicine, but the imposition of socialism throughout the economy."[30]

Health care was not to regain a leading place on the national agenda until the 1990s. In the meantime, several events bear mention:

- 1986: Congress passed the Emergency Medical Treatment and Active Labor Act (EMTALA), which requires hospitals to screen and stabilize all emergency room patients, and the Consolidated Omnibus Budget Reconciliation Act (COBRA), which allows employees to continue their group health plan (if they can afford it) up to 18 months after losing their jobs.[31]
- 1988: Congress passed the Medicare Catastrophic Coverage Act, intended to protect seniors from financial ruin because of illness, expanding Medicare coverage to an unlimited number of days, eliminating co-insurance requirements for hospitalization, and setting ceilings on patients' payments for physicians, hospitals and prescription drugs. The program was to be financed

entirely by the 33 million elderly and disabled Medicare beneficiaries themselves.[32]

- 1989: Repeal of the 1988 Catastrophic Coverage Act; a firestorm erupted across the country by angry seniors protesting their full responsibility for these new benefits in the 1988 Act, upset that more affluent seniors would have to pay for more than 80 percent of the program's costs. Much to the surprise of legislators and the AARP, which had supported the bill, Congress was forced to repeal the legislation the next year.[33]

Health care reform re-emerged during the 1992 election cycle as a high priority issue. By the early 1990s, competition had become the great hope to control increasing costs, decreased access, and variable quality in our market-based system.[34] Many hoped that a reorganized system could induce more competition within a more regulated insurance industry and lead toward universal coverage.

The year 1993 opened with a flurry of activity and renewed energy toward developing legislative proposals for universal coverage. President Bill Clinton appointed his wife Hillary Rodham Clinton as chairperson of the Health Care Task Force, which was carefully selected from the insurance industry and business, who were chiefly responsible for the problems of the existing system. Proceedings of the Task Force were held behind closed doors, and little input was sought from either the health professions or the public policy community.

After heated controversy among the Task Force members involving divisions within and between insurance and business interests, the American Health Security Act emerged in Congress as the Clinton Health Plan. It was soon joined in the legislative hopper by five other competing proposals. Four of the proposals, two Democratic and two Republican, were variants of managed competition, while the fifth was a single payer plan modeled after the Canadian system.[35]

As the battles ensued among competing stakeholders and their lobbyists, and as more specifics became known about each of the proposals, legislative support melted away for any of the plans. In 1994, the Clinton Health Plan (CHP) died in committee without getting to a floor vote. H.R. 3222 was the only proposal with bipartisan support, but not anywhere near enough for passage. In fact, the single payer proposal (H.R. 1200) attracted the largest number of supporters in Congress and was the only one to pass out of committee, but it was soon marginalized by lobbyists and ridiculed by the major corporate media as too "extreme" or "utopian."[36]

The CHP was criticized from most quarters as too complex, too expensive, and poorly conceived. It was seen as a sell-out to the private insurance industry, and dubbed by some observers as the Health Insurance Industry Preservation Act."[37] The final bill was 1,342 pages in length, and it became too confusing for the public and many legislators to understand. A political debacle for the Clinton Administration, its defeat was attributed to lack of support within the working middle class, concern about increased taxes, and growing anti-government resentment.[38]

With the exception of two incremental system changes, the failure of health care reform in 1994 put a stop to further efforts for the next 15 years. President Clinton signed legislation in 1997 creating the State Children's Health Insurance Program (SCHIP), which today covers only about one-half of American children. And in 2003 President George W. Bush signed the Medicare Prescription Drug, Improvement and Modernization Act (MMA), further privatizing the program by turning the new drug benefit over to the private sector and bringing on more overpaid private Medicare Advantage plans.[39] Neither bill significantly advanced the quest for universal coverage of affordable health care.

STAKEHOLDERS, STAKE CHALLENGERS AND THE POWER OF MONEY

Mark Peterson, a leading policy analyst and scholar in government affairs, gives us a useful way to better understand the political process and outcomes of reform initiatives. He sees competing interests in terms of *stakeholders,* who benefit from the status quo, and *stake challengers,* interests that challenge the status quo either because they do not benefit or are harmed by it. He also divides the last century into two parts in terms of the power relationships between the two groups. Before 1950, the major stakeholders in health care—the AMA, AHA, specialty organizations, and the health insurance industry—were not significantly opposed by serious stake challengers. After the 1950s, some stake challengers started to gain some leverage over reform efforts, including consumer groups, civil rights and women's groups. Political dynamics were further changed by splits among some stakeholder groups, such as the conflicting interests of large and small employers and disunity within the insurance industry.[40]

The demise of the CHP illustrates these concepts. The health insurance industry, for example, was split between large corporate insurers (the "Gang of Five"—Prudential, Metropolitan Life, Aetna, CIGNA, and John Hancock) and many hundreds of small insurers with their own trade group, the Health Insurance Association of America (HIAA). The CHP was brought down in large part by the HIAA-funded national television advertising campaign "Harry and Louise," part of a coordinated effort with other special interests vested in our market system. As actors, Harry and Louise sat down at their kitchen table to debate the CHP, concluding that it couldn't possibly work. Little did the public know that small insurers were fighting for their lives against the Gang of Five, whose agenda was to drive small insurers out of business. These internal divisions among the stakeholders themselves forced more and more compromises in Congressional committees as the "reform" proposals became more complex, lost coherence, and left the public totally confused.

LESSONS FROM A CENTURY OF FAILURES IN HEALTH CARE REFORM

This latest reform attempt may seem more successful because the resulting legislation was actually enacted into law. But the disappointing outcome could have been predicted. All five major efforts to reform our health care system over the last 100 years failed, often for similar reasons.

These lessons from history show how closely the 2009-10 effort fits historical patterns.

1. Turning to the stakeholders, who themselves created the system's problems, for recommended solutions does not work. For example, the Health Care Task Force was convened by Hillary Clinton for the CHP in an effort to gain their approval for a final legislative plan, which instead was drafted to serve their divided and separate self-interests, not the public interest, finally succumbing to its own contradictions.

The Obama Administration started negotiating deals with stakeholder industries at the onset of this latest reform effort in 2009, thereby whittling away prospects for real reform.

2. *The more complex a bill becomes, in an effort to respond to conflicting political interests, the more its legislative and public support erodes.* Compromise begets more compromise, limiting the eventual effectiveness of reform if a bill ever does get passed. The 1,342 page CHP bill could not even get out of committee in Congress. The same cumulative complexity occurred as the Obama plan moved through Congress, adding pounds to the final 2,000 plus-page Senate bill. These outcomes are in striking contrast to the successful passage of Canada's single payer plan, the Canada Health Act of 1984, defined by five basic principles—*public administration, comprehensiveness, universality, portability,* and *accessibility*—in only several pages.[41]

3. *Strong presidential leadership from the start and throughout the legislative process is critical to enactment of health care reform.* Thus, FDR could not have achieved Social Security if he had left it up to both parties in Congress. He relished the battle, and was ready from the start to pass it on a partisan basis. Consider instead what might have happened in 1993-1994 with strong presidential leadership. Dr. Quentin Young, Coordinator of Physicians for a National Health Program, asked this important question:

> "Instead of his 1,342 page monstrosity, imagine if the President supported the McDermott-Conyers-Wellstone single payer bill. With perhaps 150 votes in the House and, maybe, a dozen in the Senate, he could have faced the voters on November 8 as the champion of a People's health care plan. Is it not possible that the reactionary triumph could have been avoided? Remember, exit polls found the voters still designating health reform number one among their concerns. More importantly, would not some portion of the 61% of the electorate who didn't vote be finally moved to participate?"[42]

4. *Corporate power in our enormous medical-industrial complex, accounting for one-sixth of the nation's gross domestic product, trumps the democratic process.* The scope and power of corporate stakeholders in our largely for-profit, investor-owned market-based system have grown steadily over many years. These stakeholders and their well-paid lobbyists are expert in using the revolving door between industry, K Street and government to their own advantage and avoiding interference by government in their business interests. A huge gap in power and influence persists between stakeholders and stake challengers, with defenders of the public interest in a far weaker position. Because of that gap, we should demand that those involved in planning for reform assure that independent and non-partisan advocates of the public interest are centrally involved throughout the political process.

5. The "mainstream" media are not mainstream at all, and have conflicts of interest based on their close ties to corporate stakeholders in the status quo. As Ralph Nader points out: "[the major media conglomerates] are businesses that rely on advertising revenue and the goodwill of the surrounding business community."[43] There are many close and invisible ties between corporate health care interests and the media (e.g. General Electric, which is heavily invested in the insurance and medical industries, owns NBC;[44] CEOs of insurance companies serve on the editorial board of the *New York Times*). It is therefore no surprise that during the 1993-1994 reform attempt, there was only one mention of the single payer proposal on ABC's *"World News Tonight,"* and some TV station managers admitted their reluctance to run ads favoring single payer in order to avoid antagonizing the insurance industry.[45,46]

6. We can count on opponents to use fear mongering to distort the health care debate. The events of the last two years discussed in Chapter four have a long history in this country. Fear-mongering dates back to the first attempt to reform health care in Teddy Roosevelt's time. Jonathan Oberlander, Professor of Political Science at the University of North Carolina and author of *The Political Life of Medicare*, has noted that this pattern has existed for almost 100 years. Opponents of NHI in 1915 cast it as the nation's greatest international threat—that it "was a plot by the German emperor to take over the United States." Fast forward to the 1940s, when opponents warned that "if we adopted national health insurance, the Red army would be marching through the streets of the U.S. ... this was the first step toward communism."

Then, in the 1990s, in its opposition to the Clinton Health Plan, the health insurance industry raised doubts, through their fictional couple, Harry and Louise, how that plan might hurt the middle class rather than helping them. Oberlander sums up this long historical pattern by noting: "[T]he opponents have changed over time; the tactic of relying on fear and scaring Americans has not."[47]

7. Centrist middle of the road reform proposals for health care are bound to fail. Such proposals inevitably get watered down through the political process, responding to concerns of both the right and the left, until they are certain to be ineffective in addressing the fundamental problems calling for reform in the first place. When market stakeholders are centrally involved in planning "reforms," they will win and the public will lose. The reform proposals seriously considered by Congress in the past have not provided the voting public and its elected representatives the stark contrasts needed in reform alternatives.

8. Framing the basic issues in the health care reform debate has been inadequate; the alternatives have been controlled by the special interests resisting reform so they will win. If we were to examine the track record of the private health insurance industry over the past 40 years and compare it with single payer financing through a national system of social insurance, as almost all industrialized countries have implemented, we would find an extensive body of health policy literature that supports public financing combined with a private delivery system. As argued in my recent book, *Do Not Resuscitate: Why the Health Insurance Industry Is Dying and How We Must Replace It*, this industry is obsolete and too inefficient, expensive, unstable and unreliable to serve the public interest.[48] The fundamental question in health care reform is therefore whether or not we should retain a failing multi-payer private-public system or shift to not-for-profit public financing coupled with a private delivery system. Despite all the evidence in its favor, however, the single payer option has yet to be presented to the public as one of the main options to reform the system.

9. History repeats itself, and we don't learn from past mistakes. We have already seen a number of examples—control over framing of the alternatives by corporate stakeholders; stakeholders forcing political compromises through well-financed lobbying campaigns that gut legislation (1970s and 1990s); and a corporate media that we don't call to account for its dearth of investigative reporting and its financial conflicts of interest with stakeholders in the status quo. As we look at each of the past major attempts to reform health care, these same patterns persist through the 2009-10 reform effort even though they have been demonstrated in the past to be part of the problem. We can also see that NHI is hardly a new proposal in America—when Teddy Roosevelt brought it forward in 1912, it was no more a fringe or utopian concept than it is today.

In the next chapter we will try to take these lessons from history into account in outlining a road map to real health care reform.

References

1   Wilbur, RL. As cited in Simone, JV. Health care access, quality and economics in 1932: The eloquence of Ray Lyman Wilbur. *Oncology Times*, February 10, 2008: p. 6.

2.   Wildavsky,A. *Speaking Truth to Power: The Art and Craft of Policy Analysis.* New Brunswick, NJ: Transaction Books, 1987, p 38.

3.   Goodridge, E, Amquist, S. A history of health care reform. *New York Times*, August 17, 2009.

4.   Starr, P. *The Social Transformation of American Medicine.* New York: Basic Books, 1982.

5.   Somers, AR, Somers, HM. *Health and Health Care: Policies in Perspective.* Germantown, MD: Aspen Systems Corp, 1977.

6.   Ibid # 5.

7.   Davis, MM. The American approach to health insurance. *Milbank Q*, July 12, 1934: 214-5.

8.   Smith, JS. Roosevelt: The great divider. Op-Ed. *The New York Times*, September 3, 2009: A25.

9.   Ibid # 5.

10.   Ibid # 3.

11.   Truman, HS. A National Health Program: Message from the president. *Soc Secur Bulletin.* 1945: 8:12.

12.   Ibid # 5.

13.   Ibid # 4.

14.   Poen, M. *Harry S. Truman versus the Medical Lobby: The Genesis of Medicare.* Columbia: University of Missouri Press, 1979: 85-6.

15.   Schiltz, ME. *Public Attitudes Toward Social Security, 1935-1965.* Research report no. 33. Washington, D.C. Social Security Administration, Office of Research and Statistics, 1970: 136-9.

16.   Ibid # 15, p134.

17.   Ibid # 4.

18.   Ibid # 5.

19.   Ibid # 3.

20.   Ibid # 3.

21. Ibid # 3.
22. Michelman, F. Forward: On protecting the poor through the Fourteenth Amendment. The Supreme Court, 1968 term. *Harv L. Rev.* 1969: 83-7.
23. Kaufman, CL. The right to health care: Some cross-national comparisons and U.S. trends in policy. *Soc Sci Med.* 1981: 15(4): 157-62.
24. Ibid # 3.
25. Weaver, C. Obama's health care dilemma evokes memories of 1974. *Kaiser Health News,* September 3, 2009.
26. Ibid # 4.
27. Insuring the nation's health. *Newsweek*, June 3, 1974: 73-4.
28. Ibid # 4.
29. Ibid # 3.
30. Bartlett, B. The party of Medicare. *Forbes*, August 28, 2009.
31. Ibid # 3.
32. Ibid # 3.
33. Himmelfarb, R. *Catastrophic Politics: The Rise and Fall of the Medicare Catastrophic Coverage Act of 1988.* University Park: Pennsylvania State University Press, 1995, p 80.
34. McNerney, WJ. C Rufus Rorem Award Lecture. Big questions for the Blues: Where to go from here? *Inquiry* 33(2): 110-17, 1996.
35. Teach, RL. Health care reform: Changes and challenges. Reform teleconference draws 4,000. *Medical Group Management Update*. November 1993:4.
36. Brundin, J. How the U.S. press covers the Canadian health care system. *Int J Health Services* 23(2): 275-7, 1993.
37. Gordon, C. *The Clinton Health Care Plan: Dead on Arrival*. Westfield, NJ: Open Magazine Pamplet Series, 1995.
38. Ibid # 34.
39. Geyman, JP. *Shredding the Social Contract: The Privatization of Medicare*. Monroe, ME. Common Courage Press, 2008, p 60.
40. Peterson, M.A. Political influence in the 1990s: From iron triangles to policy networks. *J Health Polit Policy Law* 18(2): 395-438, 1993.
41. Armstrong, P, Armstrong, H. *Universal Health Care: What the United States Can Learn from the Canadian Experience*. New York: The New Press, 1998: 6-32.
42. Ibid # 37.
43. Nader, R. *Crashing the Party: Taking on the Corporate Government in an Age of Surrender*. New York: St. Martin's Griffin, 2002.
44. Hart, P, Naurecker, J. NBC slams universal health care. *EXTRA!*, December 2002: p. 4.
45. Navarro, V. Why Congress did not enact health care reform. *J Health Polit Policy Law* 20: 196-9, 1995.
46. Health Care Notes. *The Texas Observer*, December 24, 1993: 22.
47. Rovner, J. In health care debate, fear trumps logic. *NPR*, August 28, 2009.
48. Geyman, JP. *Do Not Resuscitate: Why the Health Insurance Industry Is Dying and How We Must Replace It*. Monroe, ME. Common Courage Press, 2008.

CHAPTER 12

Nobody Will Save Us But Ourselves:
A Road Map to Real Reform

"If democracy were to be given any meaning, if it were to go beyond the limits of capitalism and nationalism, this would not come, if history were any guide, from the top. It would come through citizens' movements, educating, organizing, striking, boycotting, demonstrating, threatening those in power with disruption of the stability they needed."

— Howard Zinn, author of *A People's History of the United States*[1]

"We have learned bitterly that the unlimited lobbying resources of the health industry giants can prevail in both chambers of Congress. Where, for instance, was the serious challenge from the 90 representatives on record in favor of H.R. 676, the single payer proposal? While the raucous and dangerous right-wing assault was unmitigated throughout the campaign, virtually no serious demand came from the progressive wing of the Congress. Our work is cut out for us. We have the same important challenge faced by the civil rights advocates of the 1950s and 60s, which ended victoriously. The same steady expansion of popular awareness and demand to the level of a movement is the requirement to end the current corporate control of our health system."

— Quentin Young, M.D., internist and Coordinator for Physicians for a National Health Program[2]

As we have seen in earlier chapters, the health care system is extremely complex and difficult to restructure in terms of cost control, improved access, efficiency, quality and accountability. Much of it is for-profit and investor-owned, so that the business ethic and corporate greed permeate and drive the system. The political process involved in reform attempts are even more complex, whereby corporate money drowns out the voices of the electorate.

So, now that we have a health care "reform" law, the Patient Protection and Affordable Care Act of 2010 (PPACA) that won't do the job, what can be done about it? We can start to rethink and act upon a comprehensive strategy for real health care reform. We should ignore the advice of PPACA supporters and apologists who advise us to "wait and see" how it will play out. As documented in earlier chapters, we already know how it will turn out—higher prices, higher costs, increased barriers to necessary care, worse outcomes, and greater economic hardship for many millions of Americans. The stakes are too high to wait and see.

Given all the obstacles we have seen to having an open, fair and accurate public discourse of our health care problems and policy options, can we expect a better result next time? We know there will be a next time, and it will have to come sooner than later. Despite all the hype over its potential, the PPACA will not rein in uncontrolled inflation of health care costs, either in the short or long-term. Experience over the next few years will persuade even its supporters of the naïveté of their wishful thinking.

What should we do now to build towards a victory for single payer? We can start by learning from our past mistakes, including our most recent ones as discussed in earlier chapters.

Health care reform will never be simple, since it cuts through the status quo, necessarily redistributes wealth, and impacts all parts of our society from the economic and political to the social and moral. No one legislative bill is likely to remedy our entrenched problems over financing and delivery of health care. But as a multifaceted challenge, health care reform will have to be readdressed soon, if only to avoid economic and social catastrophe.

This chapter describes essential approaches that will be required if we are to have any hope of righting the sinking health care ship.

A ROAD MAP TO HEALTH CARE REFORM:
A NINE-STEP AGENDA

The nine approaches shown in Table 12.1 will be essential elements

TABLE 12.1

A Nine-Point Approach to Real Health Care Reform

---

1. Organize for single payer public financing; abandon our multi-payer system dominated by a failing private insurance industry.
2. Demand that policy alternatives be based on credible documented health policy science and experience, not on ideology, wishful thinking, or corporate bottom lines.
3. Recognize that health care resources are limited, and must be stewarded responsibly for care of our entire population.
4. Establish an independent, non-partisan, science-based national commission to evaluate diagnostic and therapeutic interventions for comparative efficacy and cost-effectiveness, with authority to recommend coverage and reimbursement policies.
5. Change how physicians are paid.
6. Rebuild the primary care workforce.
7. Lead so the president will follow.
8. Establish majority rule in the Senate without filibuster blockade.
9. Mobilize popular support for single payer and build a social movement for real health care reform.

---

in assuring the success of health care reform the next time around.

1. Organize for single payer public financing; abandon our multi-payer system dominated by a failing private insurance industry.

The biggest single question, which if resolved could do the most to reform health care, is whether we should continue multi-payer private/public financing or adopt a publicly financed single payer system, an improved Medicare for All, coupled with a private delivery system. That option was never put on the table during this latest reform attempt.

Instead, the issues quickly became blurred in obfuscation and rhetoric disconnected from the main issues of cost, access and quality of care. The political discourse was diverted to such tangential issues as abortion and such arcane details as Exchanges and triggers. Much of the public became confused about the debate and the bills. For example, they would be wrong if they assumed that the public option (when it was even being considered) would be open to them if they were already insured and didn't like their coverage, or if they believe their employer-sponsored plans would be subject to the insurance reforms in the bills.

By contrast, widespread support for single payer financing has been documented over many decades. The single payer concept is readily understood by the electorate, especially those already covered by Medicare or counting the years until they can become eligible.

The stripped-down goals of reform should be to adopt a new system which best provides universal access to affordable, cost-effective care of good quality that is fair, sustainable and accountable. There is a mountain of evidence documenting the consistent advantages of public financing of health care in most advanced countries around the world, which policymakers and political leaders have been largely denying.

There are three general types of health care systems in the Organization for Economic Cooperation and Development (OECD) countries:

- *Single payer national health insurance (NHI) system*, with public financing of a private delivery system (e.g. Canada, Denmark, Norway, Sweden, Australia and Taiwan).
- *National health service*, with hospitals publicly owned and operated and most physicians salaried (e.g. Great Britain and Spain).
- *Highly regulated, universal, multi-payer health insurance systems*, with non-profit "sickness funds" or "social insurance funds" (e.g. Germany and France). In most of these countries, sickness funds use an "all payer" system with uniform rates for hospitals and physicians negotiated each year. These are more like "quasi-governmental agencies" that do not market, cherry pick or determine benefits. They may also provide supplementary "gap" coverage, but this amounts to less than 5 percent of health expenditures in most nations.[3]

We need to hold single payer up at one end of the spectrum to show that no other policy alternative competes against it in terms of cost, efficiency, quality, value and reliability. This option can be framed as best serving traditional American values of fairness, fiscal prudence, efficiency and accountability, and even as a patriotic way to help build a healthier population, economy and country. While single payer financing will not solve all of the system's problems directly, it will provide the structure within which to address other problems, such as negotiating prices in the public interest, reforming the reimbursement system, simplifying the administrative bureaucracy, and transitioning over time to a not-for-profit system.

As Dr. Vicente Navarro, Professor of Health Policy at The Johns Hopkins University and editor-in-chief of the *International Journal of Health Services* has observed:

> "The long history of social policy, in the U.S. and elsewhere, shows that universality is a better way to get popular support for a program than means-testing for programs targeted to specific vulnerable groups... The problem of noncoverage by health insurance will not be resolved without resolving the problem of undercoverage, because both result from the same failing: the absence of government power to ensure universal rights. There is no health care system in the world (including the fashionable Swiss model) that provides universal health benefits coverage without the government intervening, using its muscle to control prices and practices. The various proposals being put forward by the Obama administration are simply tinkering with, not resolving, the problem."[4]

2. Demand that Policy Alternatives be Based on Credible Documented Health Policy Science and Experience, not on Ideology, Wishful Thinking or Corporate Bottom Lines.

A 2009 article in *Health Affairs* documented the hazards of poor quality health policy research, noting that most health policies that are adopted are often "large-scale natural experiments with poorly understood risks and benefits." For example, when insurers add co-payments and deductibles to control spending, unintended consequences usually follow, such as reduced use of essential medications and increased costs and rates of hospitalization.[5]

As we saw in Chapter 8, the PPACA is loaded up with approaches that have already failed the tests of time and experience. These approaches were included for political reasons. Both parties were bought off with campaign contributions from corporate stakeholders in the present system. We have a law destined for failure because it succeeds wildly—for business. The quest by Democrats for bipartisanship was just a sideshow to distract from the main issue: why not single payer? The debate over policy alternatives was diverted from honest, objective assessment of their capability to address the main goals of reform— universal access, cost containment, affordability and quality.

These examples illustrate the factual disconnect between policy approaches, touted as they were, and their proven failure over many years in a number of states:

- *The individual mandate.* These have been tried by many states, including Massachusetts, California, Oregon, Pennsylvania and Maine. While expanding coverage in some situations, they have not led to cost-containment, have added to wasteful bureaucracy, have required unsustainable state subsidies, and have been plagued by premium increases by private insurers, often to the point that they exit the market.

- *The employer mandate.* The employer-based health insurance system (ESI) has been declining for many years. Established during World War II in a wartime economy, the labor market was scarce and employers attracted their workforce by offering health insurance as a key recruitment benefit. The times are now very different. Many corporate employers have outsourced jobs overseas as a means to lower their labor costs and avoid benefit coverage. Manufacturing has also gone abroad. And employers are passing on the growing costs of health insurance to their employees at an increasing rate. The ESI system has seen its best days, is an unstable and declining base for health insurance, and is obsolete. In our mobile society, young people now have an average of 11 jobs before reaching age 40. They are vulnerable to loss of insurance if they lose or change jobs, and are susceptible to "job lock" where they are forced to stay in a job they don't like just because it happens to offer health insurance.[6]

- *State high-risk pools.* These have been established by more than 30 states with the help of state and federal funding. But they cover a relatively small number of people (only about 180,000 people nationwide in 2006), and are beset by many problems, including limited benefits, high premiums and long waiting lists.[7]

- *Health insurance exchanges.* Though not a new idea, we still have no successful examples of health insurance exchanges. After sizable start-up funding, California's 15-year old Exchange was shut down in 2006. Although initially intended to enhance coverage and reduce its costs through economies of scale and market clout, none of that happened. Instead, it lacked pricing power and was burdened by adverse selection of sicker enrollees as insurers gamed the system.[8]
- *Expansion of preventive care programs in an effort to save money.* As we saw in Chapter 5, many studies (including the CBO's recent assessment) have concluded that health care costs are *increased* by expanded access to preventive services, both as a result of the costs of preventive and screening programs themselves as well as the costs of caring for the new conditions so identified.[9]

3. Recognize that health care resources are limited, and must be stewarded responsibly for care of our entire population.

Americans still have a problem acknowledging that resources are limited, although that mindset may well be changing as the recession lingers on. Many tend to think in terms of themselves, not the public good. But, as we have seen in this book, we ration care in a hard-hearted way—by ability to pay—looking the other way when so many of our fellow Americans die early or have increased hardships because of lack of access to necessary health care.

Getting back to realities, as summarized in the last chapter, we have a health care system meltdown in this country that will test our character, the real values of our society, and our democracy. And as we have seen, we can expect these realities to worsen despite the new health care bill. This brings us to a stark place—can we continue to tolerate such a cruel system wherein growing millions of our fellow Americans fall by the wayside with inability to gain access to affordable care, thereby encountering increased suffering and higher rates of preventable deaths? As the middle class continues to decline, and as gaps between the rich and the poor continue to widen, how can advantaged Americans create the health care system we all know we want?

Whenever limits are brought up through various reforms put forward to deal with this crisis, conservatives, market advocates and their allies warn us about the R word—rationing—as if we are not already doing that on the basis of ability to pay. They lead many to believe that more medical care is better, that any efforts to disturb the marketplace will ration care, that there is no need for this rich country to rein in health care prices anyway, and that free markets will fix our problems. Thus we are told to distrust scientific evidence that supports less mammography screening of low-risk women under age 50, less use of intensive hospital care for patients with no chance of recovery consistent with any quality of life, or an independent national Center for Comparative Effectiveness Research. Dean Baker, co-director of the Center for Economic and Policy Research and author of *Plunder and Blunder: The Rise and Fall of the Bubble Economy*, has this to say about the matter:

> "The insurance industry, the pharmaceutical industry, the medical supply industry and the AMA are very worried about the threat that health care reform presents to their future income. It would look unseemly for millionaires to get out in front of the public and say that we don't want health care reform because it will jeopardize our income. So instead they go into a nonsense rant about rationing."[10]

4. Establish an independent, non-partisan, science-based national commission to evaluate diagnostic and therapeutic interventions for comparative efficacy and cost-effectiveness, with the power to recommend coverage and reimbursement policies.

Shouldn't we expect that services offered in our health care system have been evaluated for efficacy, effectiveness and quality? Most patients would expect that, but we fall far short of that in our system—for many reasons, mostly tied to the financial incentives in our market-based system. Here are some of these reasons:

- About two-thirds of drug research is funded by industry, carried out in for-profit commercial research networks with much less scientific rigor than NIH studies.
- Conflicts of interest abound in relationships between industry,

researchers and their institutions over the balance of private gain vs. the public interest.

- The FDA is beholden to the drug industry for more than one-half of its annual budget.
- Negative results of studies often go unreported in the literature.
- Many studies that do get published are written by for-profit ghost-writing agencies.
- Marketing efforts are often disguised as "science."
- Past efforts to establish and maintain independent science-based federal agencies have run into political interference from lobbying by industry over "unfavorable" reviews (e.g. the former Agency for Health Care Policy and Research (AHCPR) had its funding cut and policy mission eliminated after pressure was brought on Congress by spinal surgery providers and device manufacturers in the aftermath of AHCPR guidelines favoring non-surgical approaches to low back pain.[11,12]

As we have seen in earlier chapters, up to one-third of health care services are either inappropriate or unnecessary. Peter Orszag, former CBO director, has estimated that as much as $700 billion a year could be saved if we were not paying for services lacking good clinical outcomes.[13]

It should be a no-brainer that we should establish and maintain a well-funded independent national scientific body, free from political interference, with the authority to guide health care decisions on coverage and reimbursement. We have good models for the kind of agency that is urgently needed, including the National Institute for Health and Clinical Excellence (NICE) in the United Kingdom and the Common Drug Review in Canada. If we would only do so, we should take cost-effectiveness off the third rail of health care politics and heed these sage words of Sir Michael Rawlins, chairman of NICE:

"The United States will one day have to take cost effectiveness into account. There is no doubt about it at all. You cannot keep on increasing your health care costs at the rate you are for so poor return. You are 29th in the world in life expectancy. You pay twice as much for health care as anyone else on God's earth."[14]

Unfortunately, as we have seen, the new health care "reform" law neutered the body that it will establish, the Patient-Centered Outcomes Research Institute, by denying it the power to mandate or even endorse coverage or reimbursement rules for any particular treatment.[15]

5. Change how physicians are paid.

This is absolutely essential if we are ever to have any hope of containing health care costs. Physicians order almost all health care services. We have an outdated, seriously flawed reimbursement system that dates back to the 1960s whereby most procedural services are *over*compensated while cognitive, evaluative non-procedural services are *under*compensated. Thus a primary care physician (family medicine, general internal medicine and general pediatrics) may bill about $80 for a routine office visit while an ophthalmic surgeon will bill $2,000 for a 10 or 15-minute cataract extraction. These differences have led predictably to a gross maldistribution of physicians by specialty with most medical graduates eschewing careers in primary care and instead seeking out procedural specialties offering much higher incomes and more attractive lifestyles.

As discussed earlier, it is well documented that areas with more specialists and subspecialists have the highest costs of care, typically with lower quality of care, as up to one-third of their services are either inappropriate or unnecessary. Conversely, areas with more primary care physicians have lower costs of care with higher quality.[16] Moreover, not-for-profit integrated health care systems that rely on salaried physicians, such as Kaiser Permanente and Group Health Cooperative, emphasize the provision of evidence-based care over business models that drive up the volume of services.

The PPACA makes weak attempts to deal with this issue, including delayed pilot programs to test the use of "bundled payments" and the feasibility of accountable care organizations. But most fee-for-service (FFS) reimbursement will continue for years to come, and we won't be seeing incentives to shift large numbers of physicians to salaries, especially to incomes for specialists that are less than today. Changes to the status quo will be fought fiercely by organized medicine, including the AMA and most specialty organizations, as we have already seen in the pushback by plastic surgeons over reimbursement for cosmetic procedures and radiologists over reimbursement for mammography and various imaging procedures.

Meaningful reimbursement reform should include abandonment of FFS in most settings; marked increase in the use of negotiated salaries within a publicly financed program which narrows the income gaps between specialties; expansion of group practice (even in rural areas and underserved areas, with government assistance if needed through primary care medical homes or community health centers); and disallowing reimbursement for services that are neither efficacious nor cost effective.

6. Rebuild the primary care workforce.

Nations with strong primary care systems make sure they have at least 50 percent of their physician workforce in primary care. They do this by various means, including governments picking up most of the cost of medical education, payment policies that better compensate primary care, use of salaries instead of FFS reimbursement, and some controls over funding of graduate medical education residency positions.

We have a crisis in the primary care workforce based on undersupply of providers and low reimbursement rates that leads many physicians to refuse new Medicaid and Medicare patients. This crisis will get much worse as another 30 million people gain improved access to care. The four major primary care organizations—the American Academy of Family Physicians, the American College of Physicians, the American Academy of Pediatrics, and the American Osteopathic Association— sent a letter to House and Senate leaders calling for more vigorous approaches to the primary care shortage, noting that:

> "Access to health care is more than giving someone an insurance card. It requires that patients also be able to find a primary care physician who can provide first contact, comprehensive, continuous, preventive and coordinated care for most of their health care needs."[17]

Without fundamental reimbursement reform along the lines suggested above, the renaissance of the primary care workforce to fill the needs of our population cannot occur. Given such reform, it will take many years to reach our needs, during which time these additional kinds of initiatives will be required: loan forgiveness programs for medical students entering primary care residencies; expansion of residency training programs in the primary care specialties, including support for the primary care medical home concept; and workforce policies that restrict residency positions in oversupplied specialties.

The nation needs to increase its investment in primary care if we are to rebuild the foundation of our health care system. Doubling primary care financing to 10-12 percent of total health care spending would likely pay for itself and even save money.[18] Early returns from medical home demonstrations have shown cost savings of 15 percent or more, reductions in ER visits and hospitalizations, and even lower mortality.[19]

7. Lead so the president will follow.

As we have seen, the incoming Obama administration took an overly cautious pragmatic, centrist approach intended to build a health care bill that could receive bipartisan support. President Obama waffled on many key elements, such as the public option, as he handed over the details to a widely split Congress. Health policy science was ignored from the beginning, and all the special interests that are part of the system's cost and access problem were invited to the negotiating table. This was a classic Surrender in Advance strategy that proved incapable of reforming the system. The predictable result was a bill of incremental tweaks to a failing system, a bonanza once again for the medical-industrial complex.

As we saw throughout this latest health care fight, Obama reversed himself from his earlier principled support of single payer, and kept it off the table of policy options. His campaign promises went by the board as well. He had campaigned against business as usual in Washington that allowed "lobbyists and campaign contributions to rig the system." He assured us he was "running for president to challenge that system," for "if we're not willing to take up that fight, then real change—change that will make a difference in the lives of ordinary Americans—will keep getting blocked by the defenders of the status quo." Despite these eloquent words, he did not take up that fight. As Lawrence Lessig, professor of law at Harvard Law School and co-founder of the non-profit *Change Congress* notes: "Obama will leave the presidency, whether in 2013 or 2017, with Washington essentially intact and the movement he inspired betrayed."[20]

Obama still has time to change course in his presidency. As his public approval ratings dropped below 40 percent just six months before the 2010 midterm elections, and as pundits speculated over how many seats the Republicans would pick up in Congress, he could learn from Harry S. Truman's experience in the 1948 election. Though he had an approval rating of just 33 percent in 1946, Truman saved his presidency with a comeback upset win over the heavily-favored Republican Thomas Dewey. His winning strategy was to leave the political center, rediscover his New Deal roots, and drive a consistent populist campaign that ended up as a landslide win for the Democrats, who picked up 75 seats in the House.[21]

The next time around in health care, together with a strong social movement for reform, we will need presidential leadership that takes on the corporate money-making machine of the medical-industrial complex, demands health policy evidence for the options being considered, battles for universal coverage on an equitable basis for all Americans, and sets the public interest above private gain. Obama may be more likely to pursue a course similar to Truman if we demand the change loud enough and create the political context he needs to advance a real reform agenda in health care. FDR understood this dynamic when he told activists in his own party: "I agree with you, I want to do it, now make me do it."[22]

8. Abandon the filibuster in Senate procedures in favor of majority rule.

A core democratic principle since the founding of our country has been that the majority does and should rule. Yet for many years the Senate has adopted different procedures that prevent majority rule, thus challenging the democratic process.

Filibuster is a delaying legislative maneuver dating back to the early years of Congress. The term derives from the Dutch word meaning "pirate." As the size of the House grew, it developed its own rules to limit debate, but the smaller Senate has used the filibuster on many occasions over the years. A vote to end debate by invoking cloture originally required two-thirds majority vote in the Senate, but that number was reduced to 60 in 1975. The filibuster record was established by Senator Strom Thurmond (R-SC) in 1957—24 hours and 18 minutes—in a successful effort to block the Civil Rights Act that year. This past year has seen an unprecedented increase in the use of filibuster by the minority GOP in the Senate.[23,24]

There is nothing in the Constitution about this practice. The Senate is free to establish and change its own rules. It should do so, since the nation is confronting so many large problems and needs legislative efficiency to do the people's business. Also, what's wrong with a simple majority vote anyway? As Ralph Nader counsels: "Face it—the Senate is breaking an already broken Congress into little pieces which are then sold for a mess of pottage. Organize Congress Watch Locals in every state, folks, for nobody will save you but yourselves."[25]

9. Mobilize Popular Support and
Build a Social Movement for Health Care Reform.

We know from history that transformational change of this magnitude will never happen from the top, but only from the bottom up as a sweeping social movement. That was true for women's suffrage, Social Security and civil rights, and it will be true for health care.

In spite of the partisan wrangling between the two major political parties over the future of U.S. health care, we can make a strong case that health care, as a basic human need, is different from other commodities on the open market. We all depend on access to good care whenever a medical need arises. We all confront our own personal medical crises at one or another times in our lives, and we all hope to live in a society where care will be available based on need, not cruelly rationed by ability to pay.

The health care debate is therefore not a left vs. right issue, but a top-down one. As Howard Zinn reminds us, it is the ultimate measure of a democracy:

> "Democracy is not what governments do. It's what people do. Too often, we go to junior high school and they sort of teach us democracy is three branches of government. You know, it's not the three branches of government."[26]

We have had a broad consensus in this country for some sixty years that everyone would like access to physicians, other professionals and hospitals of their own choosing within a system that is efficient, fair, sustainable and accountable for its quality. Other advanced countries have achieved all that. Why can't we join them?

Howard Zinn gives us the answer. Democracy isn't just three branches of government. Part of our problem is that we have behaved as if that's all there is to it. We've elected the right candidate—we'll probably never get anyone as clear on the virtues of single payer as Obama was *before* he became president. We've taken over the House and Senate, and Democrats will be the determining force in reshaping the judiciary as new judges are appointed. Democrats control the three branches of government, but it got us an expanded privatized disaster in health care. As Zinn tells us, democracy is something more: it requires an energized and empowered public. That is entirely up to us.

As is obvious from earlier chapters, we have an unaccountable for-profit system with runaway costs that primarily serves its corporate stakeholders, usually in conflict with the public interest. All we get is well-financed orchestrated corporate resistance, very effective whenever the status quo is threatened.

Business, both large and small, has an urgent need to contain health care costs, maintain a healthy workforce, and become more competitive in global markets. Enlightened business interests could well become a key element in a new social movement for health care reform. Businesses need efficient health care, and single payer is it. NHI will cut the costs that business is now paying for health care. NHI is for everyone; it's not a handout. It can increase rather than decrease productivity: healthy working people work harder and have lower absenteeism.

As we have seen, real health care reform has failed in every case without strong social movements from below, no matter which political party has been in power. Tommy Douglas, pioneering leader of the movement to establish single payer financing in Canada, used the following political fable, equally applicable here, to describe the failure of either party to enact reform. Here is an abbreviated version:

> Mouseland was a place where all the little mice lived and played, were born and died. And they lived much the same as you and I do. They had a Parliament and elections. They always elected a government made up of cats. The cats were nice fellows, but made laws good for cats, not mice. One law required for mouse holes to be big enough for a cat to get its paws into. Since round holes were bad, they tried square mouse holes, but they were twice as big as the round ones, and were even tougher on mice. Then they tried electing black cats, white cats, or coalitions of both. But the results were always the same until one of the mice had a better idea—elect mice instead of cats! But he was called

a Bolshevik and jailed.

Tommy Douglas always ended the story with: "But I want to remind you, you can lock up a mouse or a man but you can't lock up an idea."[27]

The Nine-Step agenda summarized in Table 12.1 (p. 235) is rational and achievable if our democracy can work, but may require other major changes before that becomes possible. Beyond what we have considered in this book, two other major barriers to the democratic process threaten to block the way forward:

- *Corporate personhood.* Corporations have been recognized as having many of the rights of persons since a landmark 1886 case before the U.S. Supreme Court—*Santa Clara County v. Southern Pacific Railroad.* Corporations were seeking protections under the law, claiming that they were "persons" who should be protected under the 14th Amendment. Although the Court did not explicitly rule on that question, corporations did gain "personhood" through an artifact of history that the Court did not actually vote on. Commenting on the case in "headnotes," J. Bancroft Davis, a former railroad executive, quoted Chief Justice Morrison Waite advising attorneys to skip arguments over whether than Amendment's equal protection clause applied to corporations since "we are all of the opinion that it does."[28] In effect that ruling was written by the railroad robber barons of the time.

  Since that time, corporations have been granted rights of free speech (to lobby their interests), Fifth Amendment protections, protection from searches, and coverage by due process and anti-discrimination laws.[29] But the biggest boon to corporate power to date came on January 21, 2010 through a horrendous decision of the U.S. Supreme Court that struck down 60 years of legal precedent prohibiting corporations from making campaign expenditures to attack or support political candidates. In *Citizens United v. Federal Election Commission,* the court ruled by a 5-4 vote that the First Amendment—designed to protect the speech of real, live human beings—guarantees for-profit corporations the right to influence elections by contributing unlimited amounts of money to campaigns.[30]

This anti-democratic decision by the Supreme Court generated an immediate firestorm of protest from many quarters, to the extent that some groups are gearing up for an effort to reverse it through a constitutional amendment that will clarify that corporations are *not* persons.

- ***Financing of elections.*** Another closely related challenge to our democracy over the last two centuries is the matter of inordinate amounts of money involved in our election process. This dates back to the first days of the Republic. In the 1850s, for example, Pennsylvania Republican Simon Cameron was promoting the "Pennsylvania Idea" of applying the wealth of corporations to help maintain Republican control of the legislature.[31]

  Many unsuccessful attempts have been tried over the years to control corporate influence over our politics. The non-partisan Center for Responsive Politics tells us that more than $560 million in campaign contributions to Congress were made through the 2008 election cycle and the first three quarters of 2009 by financial, real estate, and insurance interests. As Senator Dick Durbin (D-IL) recently said, "Frankly, the banks own the place."[32] And as lobbyist Lauren Maddox observed: "The policy process is an extension of the market battlefield."[33]

  The latest attempted fix is a bill before Congress, the Fair Elections Now Act (S. 752, H.R. 1826), which would give candidates for Congress the option to run a competitive campaign with a blend of small dollar contributions (not more than $100) and limited public funds.[34] Of course, an even more effective remedy, as so many other advanced countries have done, would be to require public financing for greatly shortened political campaigns.

Concluding Comment

These nine approaches outlined above are interdependent. Some will need to occur before single payer can be enacted. But together, in whatever sequence, they are mutually enabling as part of a coordinated progressive agenda to rein in corporate greed in deregulated health care markets and reform our system in the public interest. In the next and final chapter, we will see how the next reform effort will be different, and will finally triumph over the robber barons of our time.

References

1.   Zinn, H. as cited in Moyers, B. Howard Zinn interview. *Truthout*, December 14, 2009.
2.   Young, Q. Where we are now on health care reform. *Huffington Post*, March 30, 2010.
3.   Hellander, I. International health systems for single payer advocates. The National Health Program Reader. Leadership Training Institute. Physicians for a National Health Program, October 24, 2008.
4.   Navarro, V. Obama's mistakes in health care reform. *CounterPunch*, September 7, 2009.
5.   Majumdar, SR, Soumerai, SB. The unhealthy state of health policy research. *Health Affairs Web Exclusive* W-900-8, August 11, 2009.
6.   Weisberg, J. We are what we treat. *Newsweek*, July 18, 2009.
7.   American Diabetes Association. High-risk pools. Health Insurance Resource Manual. Alexandria, VA, 2006.
8.   Building a National Insurance Exchange: Lessons from California. Issue Brief. California HealthCare Foundation, July 2009.
9.   *ABC News*. Congressional budget expert says preventive care will raise – not cut – costs. August 9, 2009.
10. Baker, D. It's not rationing, stupid! *The Progressive Populist*, August 15, 2009: 12-3.
11. Geyman, JP. *The Corporate Transformation of Health Care: Can the Public Interest Still Be Served?* New York. Springer Publishing Company, 2004: pp 145-70.
12. Deyo, RA, Psaty, BM, Simon, G et al. The messenger under attack: Intimidation of researchers by special interest groups. *N Engl J Med* 336: 1176,1997.
13. Kaiser Daily Health Policy Report, August 4, 2008.
14. Rawlins, M. As quoted by Silberman, J. Britain weighs the social cost of high-priced drugs. *NPR*, July 3, 2008.
15. Kaiser Health News staff. True or false: Seven concerns about the new health care law. March 31, 2010.
16. Wennberg, JB, Fisher, ES, Skinner, JS. Geography and the debate over Medicare reform. *Health Affairs Web Exclusive* W-103, February 13, 2002.
17. Organizations urge Congress to strengthen primary care provisions in health care reform bills. *AAFP News Now.* December 14, 2009.
18. Phillips, RL Jr., Bazemore, AW. Primary care and why it matters for U.S.health system reform. *Health Affairs* 29:5, 806-9, 2010.
19. Grumbach, K, Bodenheimer, T, Grundy, P. The outcomes of implementing patient-centered medical home interventions: a review of the evidence on quality, access and costs from recent prospective evaluation studies [Internet]. Washington (DC): PCPCC; 2009 Aug [cited 2010 Apr 15] Available from: http://www.pcpcc.net/files/pemh_evidence_outcomes_2009.pdf.
20. Lessig, L. How to get our democracy back. There will be no change until we change Congress. *The Nation* 290 (7): 13, 2010.

21. Kuttner, R. Give 'em hell, Barry. What Barack Obama can learn from Harry Truman's inspired use of partisanship. *The American Prospect* 21 (4): 40-3, 2010.
22. Weisman, D. Now make me do it. *Political Cortex*, November 8, 2008.
23. Gill, K. Filibuster and cloture. Rules of the U.S. Senate. About.com US Politics. Accessed at http://uspolitics.about.com/od/usgovernment/a/filibuster. htm on January 5, 2009.
24. Filibuster and cloture. United States Senate. Accessed at http://www.senate. gov/artandhistory/history/common/briefing/Fi on January 5, 2009.
25. Nader, R. In the Public Interest. The filibuster flim flam. *The Progressive Populist* 15 (7): 19, April 15, 2010.
26. Ibid # 1.
27. Lingenfelter, D. The Story of Mouseland. Saskatchewan New Democrats. Accessed at http://www.saskndp.com/history/mouseland.php3 on January 4, 2010; full copy of this fable is available through that source.
28. Cullen, JM. Reject corporate personhood. *The Progressive Populist*, October 15, 2009.
29. Derber, C. *Corporation Nation: How Corporations Are Taking Over Our Lives and What We Can Do About It.* New York. St. Martin's Press, 1998, pp 4-5.
30. Weisman, R. Corporate focus. Shed a tear for democracy. *The Progressive Populist* 16 (3): February 15, 2010: p 13.
31. History of campaign finance reform. Wikipedia. Accessed January 6, 2010 at: http://en.wikipedia.org/wiki/Campaign_finance_reform.
32. Nyhart, N. Dodd's retirement is indictment of campaign finance reform. *Huffington Post*, January 8, 2010.
33. Maddox, L. As cited by Reich, R. Everyday corruption: The policy-making process has become an extension of the market battlefield. The American Prospect 21 (6): 26, July/August 2010.
34. Ibid # 32.

CHAPTER 13

Single Payer NHI:
The Only Financing System that Will Work

"If something cannot go on forever, it will stop."

—Herbert Stein, Ph.D., conservative economist, former chairman,
Council of Economic Advisors under Presidents Nixon and Ford[1]

"This is a perilous moment. The individualist, greed-driven free-market ideology that both our major parties have pursued is at odds with what most Americans really care about. Popular support for either party has struck bottom, as more and more agree that growing inequality is bad for the country, that corporations have too much power, that money in politics has corrupted our system, and that working families and poor communities need and deserve help because the free market has failed to generate shared prosperity—its famous unseen hand has become a closed fist."

—Bill Moyers, veteran journalist and commentator, and
Michael Winship, senior writer on *Bill Moyer's Journal* on PBS[2]

The 2010 health care reform law is unsustainable. It will break the bank for government payers and end up as a temporary illusion of reform that the public will see through down the line. Stein's Law quoted above will apply here. Just because our market-based system of health care has a long history does not mean it is immortal.

After this tumultuous health care debate and legislative effort to get the new law in place, it would be easy to think that reform is over for at least another decade or more. Easy—but wrong. Many on the right are waiting for an opportunity to repeal the law. Some corporate stakeholders still oppose the law while others continue lobbying against those provisions they see as onerous to their interests. On the other side, many liberals and progressives are still unhappy that the law falls too far short of reform to be acceptable. So the debate and lobbying grind on and will play a major role in the 2010 elections.[3]

One might also think that real health care reform can never pass through the U.S. Congress given the enormous political power and corporate money that stand in the way, and the lack of success of now six major attempts over the last century. Again—understandable, but shortsighted.

The 2010 political settlement over health care is flawed at its core—it simply won't work to correct the growing system problems of cost, affordability, access and quality of care. It will do the most on the access side, but only by bailing out a floundering insurance industry that will game the new system for its own profits and leave many tens of millions of Americans seriously *underinsured* along the way.

This chapter has two goals: (1) to review some of the major reasons that our present multi-payer financing system of health care *must be replaced* by not-for-profit single payer NHI; and (2) to outline many ways in which we all can participate in a growing social movement to make that happen sooner rather than later.

WHY SINGLE PAYER IS OUR BEST SOLUTION

These are some of the main reasons the country will have to adopt single payer NHI as the *only* way to save its health care system and meet its basic mission to provide the best possible care, within limited resources, to all Americans:

1. The private insurance industry can't meet the public's needs.

Despite its current political power and war chest of profits, the industry's Foundation is built on sand, quickly eroding at that. It may enjoy a short-term reprieve as a result of the 2010 bill, but only through the largesse of increased government subsidies for the individual mandate. It has become dependent on government subsidies to stay alive. The long-term outcome is obvious—*its business plan is in direct conflict with the public interest, and cannot be sustained.* Government and taxpayers will not be able to subsidize the industry indefinitely.

The following examples indicate that the industry's limited future is well known to insiders:

- Wendell Potter, long-term Cigna executive and director of communications, became a whistle-blower of the industry's many deceptive practices, including dumping of enrollees when they got sick and less profitable and "benefit design flexibility" in marketing "limited benefit plans" of little value. In testimony before Congressional committees, he came out strongly for the public option as an essential counter to the industry, much to the industry's chagrin. He ended up supporting some of the provisions of PPACA as better than no action at all, but called the new law "a joke, and an absolute gift to the industry."[4]

- At a large 2010 meeting of health economists at the Federal Reserve Bank in Chicago, addressing *New Perspectives on Health and Health Care Policy*, there was complete agreement among the participants that the private insurance industry "does not add value—they could but they do not"; when that statement came up, nobody questioned it. That was just common knowledge.[5]
- William Pewen, former senior health policy advisor for Senator Olympia Snowe (R-ME), states: "When Congress next attempts reform, in a decade or more, health costs and the number of uninsured and underinsured will have escalated—and the likely outcome will be the single payer system that Republicans most abhor."[6]
- While still profiteering through high margins and declining amounts of premium revenue going to patient care, the industry is not investing in how to provide better coverage for patients. Quite the opposite—it is maneuvering to get around restraints of the new health care bill. Even more telling as to their real motivation: insurers are buying back shares as another way to boost profits. They expect to make a great deal of money on the "reform" bill. The current price of their stock is cheap and a good investment compared to what they anticipate in gaining large new markets. This approach, of course, serves the interests of top executives by concentrating their ownership in an already consolidated industry, as well as the interests of shareholders, but doesn't add to the value of coverage for patients. In March 2010, WellPoint Chief Financial Officer Wayne DeVeydt told investors the company plans to spend almost $4 billion on share repurchases that year, compared to $2.6 billion in 2009.[7] That's $4 billion of our premium dollars we have spent trying to get

medical coverage.

2. The employer-sponsored insurance (ESI) system is continuing its long decline.

ESI is another part of the collapsing deck of cards in multi-payer financing of health care. It has been steadily unraveling for the last 60 years as the nation's economy and workforce have changed dramatically. Employers have had increasing difficulty dealing with soaring health care costs beyond their control. Only about three in five workers are now covered by their employer, and that fraction drops every year. Many employers have dropped coverage, while most have passed more and more costs along to their employees.[8]

As we have seen in earlier chapters, much of the business community does not see relief from their cost burdens in the 2010 health care legislation. Employer mandates place increased cost burdens on business, and can become an incentive for some to move out of state or even out of the country. More than one-third of the nation's employers—38 percent—will face federal penalties if their coverage is considered "unaffordable" by PPACA's requirement that employees pay no more than 9.5 percent of their household income for coverage. Employers will also be required to pay additional penalties under a "shared responsibility" provision requiring them to provide affordable coverage to part-time employees working more than an average of 30 hours per week in a month.[9] Small employers will benefit through government subsidies, but for how long?

The vulnerability and unreliability of ESI as a way to finance health care in the U.S. is revealed by a May 2010 report in *Fortune* magazine. Internal documents reviewed by *Fortune* from companies such as AT&T, Deere and others found that many large companies, in the aftermath of PPACA, are considering dumping their ESI in exchange for paying the penalties to the government. That would dismantle employer-based coverage that goes back to the 1940s, and render worthless the Democrats' promise that people could keep their insurance if they like it. AT&T produced a PowerPoint slide entitled "Medical Cost Versus No Coverage Penalty." A report prepared by Hewitt Resources, a consulting firm for Verizon, stated: "Even though the proposed assessments [on companies that do not provide health care] are material, they are modest when compared to the average cost of health care," and that to avoid costs and regulations, "employers may consider exiting the health care market and send employees to the Exchanges."[10]

3. Incrementalism that builds on our multi-payer, market-based system has not been able to control health care costs over the past 30 years, and won't do so in the future.

There is widespread agreement that the 2010 health care legislation will not control escalating costs of care. True, a few gimmicks were thrown in toward the end of this decade as gestures in that direction, such as tweaks in changing how physicians are paid and untested accountable care organizations. But these will not put a dent in the crushing bills of patients, families and payers. Les Funtleyder, a health care analyst at Miller Tabak, an institutional brokerage firm and asset manager, commented: "There does not seem to be any onerous cost control."[11]

The PPACA pulls out all of the failed incremental approaches of past years, offering them up as somehow more effective this time. We have seen employer and individual mandates before in many states, as well as failed promises for prevention and wellness programs, disease management, information technology and the rest. The hybrid "reform" plan enacted in Massachusetts in 2006—a template for the PPACA—is already failing on cost control. The state's health care costs rose by 15 percent, twice the national average, from 2006 to 2008, and the state has already started to cut back on coverage.[12] There are no silver bullets for the present system.

We need more fundamental reform. Shifting to a not-for-profit public system of financing a private delivery system will automatically open up otherwise unavailable ways to improve access (universal access overnight without cost-sharing), cost containment (global budgeting, negotiated prices and fees, bulk purchasing, reduced administrative costs) and quality (reduction of disparities, evidence-based coverage and reimbursement policies, more system accountability).

Health information technology (HIT) gives us one example of how single payer NHI will provide the structure within which to make needed changes. A 2009 national study of about 4,000 U.S. hospitals, including those on a list of the "100 Most Wired," found no evidence that HIT lowered costs or streamlined administration. In fact, the most wired hospitals had the largest increases in administrative costs. U.S. hospitals maintain administrative costs of about 25 percent, double that of their Canadian counterparts. By contrast, the HIT success story is with our VA system, which as a single payer system uses global budgets, eliminates most billing and internal cost accounting and focuses its budget on actual delivery of care.[13] Beyond their administrative efficiency, VA hospitals have demonstrated over many years better quality of care compared to civilian hospitals.[14]

4. Business may revolt if it finally decides that it can't contain its health care costs without single payer.

It still surprises me that business has been so slow in recognizing that a deregulated health care market is its unmanageable and unsustainable albatross. A few voices in big business have recognized the problem for some years, but they are in the minority. Here is what the vice chairman of Ford Motor Company had to say in 2004:

> "[High health care costs have] created a competitive gap that's driving investment decisions away from the U.S… Right now the country is on an unsustainable track and it won't get any better until we begin—business, labor and government in partnership—to make a pact for reform. A lot of people think a single payer system is better."[15]

But the day is not far off when business—big and small—will unite in favor of a more efficient, less expensive way to assure a healthy workforce that will give them the opportunity to compete more effectively in global markets. Edward Luce, Washington Bureau Chief for the *Financial Times*, has this to say:

> "…in terms purely alone of American competitiveness, …just in terms of putting a lid on the galloping costs in the American economy, the disincentive to creating a new manufacturing job here for example, as opposed to in China, or Canada for that matter, I would have a single payer system. A single payer system would be able to negotiate like a monopsony, which is the buyer side of a monopoly, and to reduce drug prices which is one of the biggest contributors to health care inflation in America. It would be able to do all sorts of things to drive health care costs down, and would help to solve America's fiscal problem."[16]

We have seen earlier how the business community is already showing cracks in its solidarity. This is the National Federation of

Independent Business' view of the Senate bill just before the passage of health care "reform" on March 21, 2010:

> "The road to ruin is paved with good intentions. The Senate health care bill is filled with good intentions. It shares many of the weaknesses of state-level reforms that failed catastrophically in recent years... The pattern looks something like this: The state enacts reforms designed to expand coverage. The reforms do little to push costs down, yet supporters assume that savings will materialize at some unspecified future date. The coverage expansion alters incentives, in turn undermining the stability of private insurance pools and pushing people into public programs. As a result, private insurance markets crumble and the government's financial burden soars. Unable to bear the burden, the state government eventually repeals the reforms and renounces its earlier promises. Some individuals lose their insurance coverage. The system never fully recovers."[17]

Business and the public share the same interests when it comes to health care. Both want full access to efficient, affordable health care of good value and quality. They are on the same side in this desire. As their health care costs become even more onerous under PPACA, we can expect the business community will see the advantages of universal coverage under single payer NHI which will cost them less than they are paying now.

5. Labor may also revolt when it sees more clearly that affordable health care is becoming even more elusive.

The PPACA does not prevent employers from continuing to shift more costs of insurance and health care to their employees. Some employers will still drop coverage and pay whatever penalty becomes required by the government. People losing coverage will not be eligible for coverage through the Exchanges until 2014, and even then may not be able to afford it.

Organized labor has become increasingly vocal in its support for single payer in recent years. At its national conference in 2009, for example, the AFL-CIO passed Resolution 34 unanimously, which states in part:

> "Universal health care does not mean mandating that everyone

must buy a health insurance policy and then handing them the bills." David Newby, president of the Wisconsin State AFL-CIO, adds: "Achieving Medicare for All is critical to the future of the labor movement. Our movement is growing because the proposed national reforms fall far short of the health security that all workers need. Our economic future depends on making the right policy choices on health care—and that's single payer."[18]

We can expect labor's support for single payer will only become stronger and more united in the next few years as labor sees how little the 2010 bill helps them.

6. State and federal governments will not be able to sustain their increasing burdens of health care costs as the safety net further deteriorates and other priorities intervene.

As the most serious recession since the 1930s continues, government coffers at all levels are being stressed to the hilt. The following are examples of just how dire the current circumstances are for states, even before the planned expansion of Medicaid in 2014:

- According to a new report from the Pew Center on the States, state governments are confronting at least a trillion dollar gap between the health care, pension and other retirement benefits promised to public employees and the money allocated for them.[19]
- Raymond Scheppach, head of the National Governors Association, says that states face a "lost decade" due to falling tax revenues and a "broken fiscal model" exposed by the recession.[20]
- As they face relentless fiscal pressures, almost all states are considering cuts in Medicaid, especially by cutting "optional benefits" such as vision and dental care, and cutting payments to physicians and other health professionals.[21]
- In Los Angeles County, reimbursement rates for emergency room physicians and on-call specialists were cut from 27 percent to just 18 percent of estimated fees for the first three days of care at private hospitals under the Physician Services for Indigents Program; more than one-half of the County's 72 hospitals are operating at a deficit, two are in bankruptcy, and 11 have closed since 2002.[22]

- In Arizona, the governor's 2011 budget will drop 300,000 people off of state health care programs, including elimination of KidsCare, which provides health care to nearly 40,000 children of low-income parents.[23]
- In Michigan, many Medicaid benefits have been eliminated, including dental, vision, podiatry, hearing and chiropractic services, and reimbursement rates have been cut for physicians to little more than comparable reimbursement under Medicare. Many physicians will no longer see Medicaid patients. In Genesee County, the birthplace of General Motors, one in four non-elderly residents are uninsured, and another one in five is on Medicaid.[24]

The situation is also serious at the federal level. In the coming decade 2009-2019, the Office of the Actuary of CMS estimates that health care spending will grow by an average of 6.1 percent annually, a rate well in excess of inflation. In 2010, national health expenditures (NHE) were more than $2.5 trillion, accounting for 17.3 percent of the GDP and averaging $8,231 per capita. The economic recession and rising unemployment are among the factors that will drive up health care costs in this coming decade. *Public* spending on health care is expected to consume more than one-half of all U.S. health care spending by 2012.[25] But as we know, those figures are only for *federal* health care spending, not the total spending on health care that patients and families have to pay. And these figures are grossly understated because they leave out two other important taxpayer sources of health care financing— tax subsidies through tax deductions for ESI plans, and subsidies for the purchase of health benefit programs for public employees, which together account for about another 15 percent of federal spending on health care. So the real figure is that the government pays about two-thirds of our total NHE.[26]

The health care law, projected to cost $1 trillion over the next ten years, will likely cost much more. As we recall, about one-half of that amount was allocated to pay for the bill, partly from "savings," which will probably not materialize, or actual cuts in Medicare spending, which may not be politically acceptable when it comes down to it. The Office of the Actuary projects that the NHE share of the GDP will reach 21 percent in 2019, more than the 20.8 percent under prior law.[27]

David Sirota, progressive blogger (OpenLeft.com) and author of the 2008 book, *The Uprising: An Unauthorized Tour of the Populist Revolt Scaring Wall Street and Washington*, correctly describes the new health care law as "a liberal wager that Medicaid plus subsidies will equal universal health care." But he notes the obvious pitfall that its soaring costs, without effective regulation, will "turn the Treasury into an unlimited gift card for whichever private interests are being sponsored."[28]

And as we saw in Chapter 10, the enormous continuing growth in health care inflation is the driving force that will make for intolerable deficits in the future. This is not mainly because of overutilization of our health care system, as conservatives like to think, but because the prices of health care commodities in the U.S. are virtually uncontrolled.[29]

7. Support for NHI is growing among physicians and other health professionals.

Physicians and other health care professionals provide all of our health care. Employers, hospitals, drug companies and other of the many corporate parts of the medical industrial complex do not. But unfortunately, physicians and other health professionals have lost much of their control over how medicine is practiced, beholden as they increasingly are as employees of larger systems.

Predictably, a growing proportion of physicians and other health professionals are fed up with the expanding bureaucracy of our complex and dysfunctional multi-payer financing system, which will only get more burdensome as the new health care "reform" bill plays out. They are realizing that under single payer NHI, they would have more time and energy for direct patient care, simplified billing with lower practice overhead, more clinical autonomy with less hassle from clerks in multiple insurance plans, and more predictable income. All patients would be "paying patients," and physicians would no longer have to worry about their patients not gaining access to needed care.

We can expect that physicians and other health professionals will take a more activist role in advocacy for their patients, even to the point of protests and potential short work stoppages to get the attention of policymakers, politicians, media and the public. Activist positions for single payer NHI have already been taken by some professional organizations, including the American College of Physicians (ACP, the second largest organization of physicians in the country with 125,000 members), Physicians for a National Health Program (PNHP), the American Public Health Association (APHA), and the California Nursing Association (CNA). A 2008 study of more than 2,200 U.S. physicians in 13 specialties found that 59 percent support NHI; with the exception of three specialties—surgery, anesthesiology and radiology, all at the higher end of the reimbursement spectrum—more than 50 percent of all the other specialties favored NHI.[30]

8. We can expect a strong backlash from a growing part of the population that begins to understand that the new health care "reform" law won't make them any better off, and in fact will leave many worse off.

We have been told from the beginning that we can keep our insurance if we like it, and that the combined employer/individual mandate in a subsidized multi-payer system will expand access to 94 percent while making us all better off. As we have seen in earlier chapters, this is far from the truth. There are many ways in which people can lose their coverage, and not regain adequate coverage once lost. Future experience with PPACA will probably show that assurances to the contrary are simply snake oil.

Our already complicated and dysfunctional system just got more so. Many people will still lose coverage if their employers drop it or make it unaffordable through increased cost-sharing. Exchanges won't be up and running for four years, and the question then will be whether people can afford coverage, and how much value that would mean as health care prices continue to skyrocket. Expanded Medicaid is also four years away, and by then its coverage is likely to be even more barebones than it is today. Dr. Don McCanne, senior health policy fellow at PNHP, sums up the problem this way:

> "People already understand that health care costs are too high. What they need to understand is that they cannot rely on being able to keep the insurance they have if it becomes unaffordable for themselves or their employers, and they cannot rely on being able to purchase it through an exchange if the premiums are too high and subsidies are too low. They also need to understand that, even if they have insurance, the relatively low actuarial value of basic coverage will leave them exposed to financial hard-

ship should they develop significant health care needs, so the insurance they have won't work as it should."[31]

A Kaiser Health Tracking poll in April 2010, about a month after passage of the health care bill, found that 55 percent of respondents were confused about the legislation. When asked how they thought it would impact themselves and their families, the results were split evenly—three in ten felt they would be better off, while the same number felt they would either be worse off or make no difference.[32] Of course, we can anticipate that both major political parties will attempt to persuade the electorate to their side of the story, but there is not likely to be widespread public support for the reform law, especially as more people become aware of its shortcomings.

9. We ignore lessons from health care systems in other advanced countries at our peril.

Our health care system continues as "odd man out" among health care systems around the world. We think we have the best system–but we don't. As we have seen, many other nations outperform the U.S. on virtually every measure of care except cost. Here we really are the world leader, with no end to health care inflation in sight.

The Democrats have bought into the illusion that we can control health care prices and costs by maintaining our multi-payer, largely for-profit private financing system with very little regulation. This is a dream that will turn into a nightmare. There is no country in the world that can achieve universal coverage while leaving some role for private insurers, without requiring them to function as not-for-profits under heavy government regulation.[33]

Lessons from abroad should teach us that we cannot achieve universal access and cost containment without a strong role by a government committed to assuring affordable access to necessary care for all Americans. Access without cost and price controls is doomed to failure, especially in a market-based system that remains relatively deregulated.

The health care "reform" bill has given the corporate foxes free rein of the hen house, and will turn out to be better for Wall Street and the medical industrial complex than the middle class and Main Street.

As we enter the political battles in the 2010 election cycle, the appropriate role and size of government is hotly debated, but with little accuracy. Republicans argue for small government but have built big government over the last 30 years. Republican candidates are courting the senior vote by disingenuosly posturing as defenders of Medicare,[34,] an entitlement program they have wanted to see "wither on the vine" ever since the Gingrich-led 1994 Contract with America.[35] Conservatives want to keep corporate-friendly government policies in place while retaining free market policies. The financial industry is trying to buy its way to less reform than Main Street would like to see.[36]

Health care "reform" is more an example of corporate welfare than of making health care affordable for everyone. The real question we should be debating, as Howard Zinn reminds us, is: "Big government in itself is hardly the issue. The question is: Whom will it serve? Or rather, which class?"[37]

Conservatives in this country rail against the specter of "socialized medicine," but they could learn from the recent elections in the United Kingdom. The new Conservative Leader David Cameron became Prime Minister in May 2010, after his party had been out of power for thirteen years. Twenty votes short of a majority, he put together an alliance with the Liberal Democrats to form the first coalition government since World War II.[38] Throughout the election campaign, there was full support for the National Health Service (NHS) across the entire political spectrum. Enacted in 1948, it was viewed as sacrosanct. The Conservative Party calls itself "the party of NHS." As Prime Minister Cameron acknowledges on his party's web site:

> "Millions of people are grateful for the care they have received from the NHS – including my own family. One of the wonderful things about living in this country is that the moment you're injured or fall ill – no matter who you are, where you are from, or how much money you've got – you know that the NHS will look after you."[39]

WHAT CAN WE ALL DO NOW? A CALL TO ACTION

The Challenges

Corporate stakeholders, their allies and lobbyists have won the day with this "reform" bill. The insurance industry will see tens of millions of new enrollees, many subsidized by the government, with many ways remaining to game the system, force sicker patients on to public programs, and raise premiums to what the traffic will bear. Most insurance "reforms" are largely cosmetic, and most Americans are ineligible for a weak insurance exchange. The drug and medical device industries will have to pay some new fees, but preserve their pricing prerogatives and still have industry-friendly regulation through the FDA, much of whose budget they provide. Employers will pass along more of their health care costs to their employees, and reform of physician reimbursement is still years in the future. Total health care costs for patients and their families will continue to soar at rates far higher than their incomes or the cost of living. So the final score is Medical-Industrial Complex:1, the Public Interest: 0.

Given the obstacles of health care reform as once again demonstrated over the last year, are there reasons to be optimistic about ever achieving real reform? The answer is a resounding Yes!— for a number of reasons. The first reason for optimism is that what we are left with will not work to contain health care costs, and is not sustainable. Health care continues on a path that will bankrupt many Americans, overwhelm government budgets at all levels, and hollow out our society as it becomes even more inequitable than today.

The next opportunity to re-address health care reform must come sooner rather than later. Some 150 years ago, Ralph Waldo Emerson had this to say about our need to educate ourselves and work for needed reforms:

> "Politics is an after work, a poor patching. We are always a little late. The evil done, the law is passed, and we begin the uphill agitation for repeal of that of which we ought to have prevented the enacting. We shall one day learn to supersede politics by education."[40]

Just over 20 years ago, Congress was forced by a firestorm of protest among seniors to repeal its Medicare Catastrophic Care bill a year after its passage in 1988, much to the embarrassment of Congress and the White House.[41] Flawed legislation *can* be reversed, sometimes very quickly!

The 2010 midterm elections give us a chance to keep building our base of activists for real health care reform. We already know that many millions of Americans across the entire political spectrum are opposed, for different reasons, to the health care law that Congress and the president have given us. If we mobilize an energized and educated public around the inadequacies of this bill to contain costs and make health care affordable for ordinary Americans, we can start to build strong support for doing the job right.

The basic issue is about private gain vs. the public good. Two observations some two centuries apart are relevant to this issue:

- Alexis de Tocqueville, French political thinker, historian and author of *Democracy in America*, argued in the early 19th Century that "if everyone feels the obligation to maintain a civil society, to act in a trustworthy way, and to volunteer for the nation in times of attack, then all citizens can benefit from these traditions and norms. And the benefit to one person does not reduce the benefit for others."[42]
- Henry Giroux, Global TV Network chair in the Department of English at McMaster University and author of the new book *Politics After Hope: Barack Obama and the Crisis of Youth, Race, and Democracy*, brings this current perspective to the problem:

  "Without an urgent reconsideration of the crucial place of public values in the shaping of American society, the meaning and gains of the past that extend from the civil rights movement to the antiwar movements of the '60s will be lost, offering neither models nor examples of struggles forged in the heat of reclaiming democratic values, relations and institutions."[43]

The problems at the root of our failing health care system have parallels in many other parts of our economy and society. Much as Wendell Potter, an insider with a long career in the private health insurance industry, and author of the excellent book, *Deadly Spin: An Insurance Company Insider Speaks Out on How Corporate PR is Killing Health Care and Deceiving Americans,* has blown the whistle on that industry's exploitive practices, so too have others taken up the battle to reclaim our democracy against corporate domination. The recent book by John Perkins, *Hoodwinked: An Economic Hit Man Reveals Why the World Financial Markets Imploded—and What We Need to Do to Remake Them*, reveals how corporate greed, mismanagement and deceptive practices over the last several decades have led to today's global economic meltdown. He offers us ways to take back our democracy through a socially and politically energized citizenry. As he suggests:

> "Whether you are a student, dentist, plumber, housewife, or something else, you can talk to your friends, family, and clients about the issues, join organizations that represent your passions, send e-mails, use materials that are environmentally and socially responsible, support politicians who take actions oriented to benefit future generations, vote in the marketplace for companies committed to doing the right thing, and accomplish objectives you have dared only dream about until now... You too can change the world. Commit to honoring your passion and acknowledging your power."[44]

Some Concrete Ways to Become an Activated Change Agent

Chris Hedges reminds us that "social change is delivered through activism, organizing and mobilization that empower groups to confront the hegemony of the corporate state and the power elite."[45] And Samuel Adams, statesman, political philosopher and one of our Founding Fathers, had this to say more than two centuries ago: "It does not require a majority to prevail, but rather an irate, tireless minority keen to set brush fires in people's minds."[46]

Here are some concrete ways in which every one of us can become an activated change agent towards building a powerful social movement for real health care reform:

1. Educate yourself on the issues.

This is now easier than ever before. We know what the problems are, how incremental reforms have failed and will do so again, and we have excellent educational resources available through such organizations as Physicians for a National Health Program (www.pnhp.org), the California Nurses Association (www.calnurses.org), and Healthcare-NOW! (www.healthcare-now.org). There is also a growing body of authoritative progressive sources of information on the airwaves and in the print media, including *Democracy Now!*, (which airs on more than 800 TV and radio stations worldwide), radio shows by Ed Schultz and Stephanie Miller, *The Nation*, *The Progressive*, the *Progressive Populist*, AlterNet, Public Citizen, and Fairness and Accuracy in Reporting (FAIR).

2. Communicate your concerns widely, whether by talking, public speaking, writing letters and op-eds, email or other ways.

We are seeing incredible advances in social networking facilitated by new technologies. In their excellent recent book *Connected: The Surprising Power of Our Social Networks and How They Shape Our Lives*, Nicholas Christakis and James Fowler show us how effective social networking can be in restoring our democratic process through their *Three Degrees Rule*. By one degree of separation, they mean our communications with friends; two degrees involves the friends of our friends, and three degrees our friends' friends' friends. Based on an assumption that we communicate with 20 people at each of the three degrees of separation, they build a reasonable argument that an energized citizen can influence as many as 8,000 people in this way![47]

3. Select a part of the health care reform agenda to focus on that best fits your interests, passion and situation.

With single payer NHI as the goal, we need to change the political landscape to force Congress and the president to enact it. Anything that contributes to this is important, whether it's by writing to your congress person, demonstrating or contacting local businesses to take a stand. As we saw in the last chapter, success in real health care reform will require a coordinated effort along several lines of attack. But that may also require other steps, such as passage of Fair Elections legislation, campaign finance reform with teeth, a constitutional amendment to repeal the latest decision by the U.S. Supreme Court on corporate campaign contributions as their "free speech," and public financing of elections. So pick your area, educate yourself in that area, and join whatever organized groups are spearheading that change. Examples include:

- For single payer NHI :
  www.singlepayeraction.org,
  www.laborforsinglepayer.org,
  www.unionsforsinglepayer.org, and
  www.calnurses.org.
- Fair Elections Now Act, a bill sponsored by Senator Richard Durbin (D-IL) and Representative John Larson (D-CT), that would provide Congressional candidates with an alternative to corporate-funded campaigns before fundraising for the 2010 elections is in full swing.
- Americans before Corporations amendment:
  www.movetoamend.org,
  www.freespeechforpeople.org, and
  www.dontgetrolled.org
- Public financing and campaign finance reform
  www.commoncause.org, and
  www.publiccampaign.org.

4. Work with state-based single payer groups and support progressive initiatives and referenda.

Opportunities are increasing for activists to work with state-based single payer initiatives in a number of states. Vermont has passed a law mandating design of new health care models, including single payer. Other states have introduced similar bills, including California, Minnesota, Ohio and Maryland.

The Ballot Initiative Strategy Center has emerged as the chief proponent of employing initiatives and referenda to advance progressive policies. Its 2009 report, *Ballot Integrity: A Broken System in Need of Solutions*, led to media attention of fraudulent petitioning placing issues on state and local ballots, legal recourse and legislative remedies.[48]

5. Join the divestiture movement to counter rapacious corporate theft of our affordable health care for their own shareholders and CEOs.

Progressive activists have developed a shareholder resolution, to be presented at the 2010 annual meeting of Anthem/WellPoint in Indianapolis, that calls on the Board of Directors to launch a feasibility study to return to not-for-profit status, thereby eliminating ownership interests of shareholders. Although the company will oppose that resolution, activists are planning a further strategy to build a national divestiture movement against those many corporations that exploit the public interest for their own profits. Contacts are being made with Consumers Union in California and the Socially Responsible Investing community (SRI).[49]

6. *Vote double-talking politicians out of office.*

We have seen many examples of politicians in both parties who for years have talked out of both sides of their mouths on specific issues. The health care battle of 2009-10 has many examples, as we have seen. This has led a large part of the electorate to growing distrust of the government, a serious handicap when government should be part of the solution to many of our problems. We need to hold all of our political leaders accountable for their behavior, not their words, and vote them out of office when they skirt the public interest.

We, the Public, Have Power We Haven't Used Yet

As Americans, we have made big course changes and improved our society in the past, as witnessed by women's suffrage, civil rights and ending a losing war in Vietnam. It is now time to step up to the health care challenge. There's a win-win result for everyone if we can develop the political will and power of a re-energized democracy to reform our health care system. Future generations are counting on us.

These eloquent words of Howard Zinn, who died in 2010 after a distinguished career as a scholar, historian and political activist for the common good, inspire us to the coming battles over health care and our democracy:

"To be hopeful in bad times is not foolishly romantic. It is based on the fact that human history is a history not only of cruelty, but also of compassion, sacrifice, courage, kindness. What we choose to emphasize in this complex history will determine our lives. If we see only the worst, it destroys our capacity to do something.

If we remember those times and places—and there are so many—where people have behaved magnificently, this gives us the energy to act, and at least the possibility of sending this spinning top of a world in a different direction. And if we do act, in however small a way, we don't have to wait for some grand utopian future. The future is an infinite succession of presents, and to live now as we think human beings should live, in defiance of all that is bad around us, is itself a marvelous victory."[50]

References

1. Stein, H. As quoted in Wikipedia, accessed April 18, 2010.
2. Moyers, B, Winship, M. Dr. King's economic dream deferred. *Truthout*, April 3, 2010.
3. Fram, A. The influence game: Health care fight still rages. Associated Press, April 17, 2010.
4. Potter, W. Public option essential, Baucus plan an "absolute gift" to health insurance industry. Huffington Post, November 15, 2009.
5. Hellander, I, personal communication, April 12, 2010.
6. Pewen, WF. The health care letdown. *New York Times*, March 15, 2010.
7. Berry, E. Health plan profits: Relying on the market. *American Medical News*, April 5, 2010.
8. Taylor, H. How and why the health insurance system will collapse. *Health Aff (Milwood)* 21: 195, 2002.
9. Mercer. A third of employers may be penalized for health coverage deemed 'unaffordable'. April 27, 2010.
10. Tully, S. Documents reveal AT&T, Verizon, others thought about dropping employer-sponsored benefits. *Fortune*, May 6, 2010.
11. Fabrikant, G. Health care overhaul may help a fund sector. *New York Times*, April 9, 2010.
12. Himmelstein, DU, Woolhandler, S. Obama's reform: no cure for what ails us. *British Medical Journal* 340: 1778, 2010.
13. Mearian, L. Harvard study: Computers don't save hospitals money. *ComputerWorld*, November 30, 2009.
14. Arnst, C. The best medical care in the U.S. *Business Week*, July 17, 2006.
15. Downey, K. A heftier dose to swallow. *Washington Post*, March 6, 2004.
16. Luce, E. C-SPAN. Washington Journal, April 30, 2010. Available at http://www.cspan.org/Watch/Media/2010/04/30/WJE/R32382/Friday+April+30.aspx.
17. National Federation of Independent Business. To Congress: Three proverbs for healthcare reform. March 18, 2010.
18. Kosuth, D. Labor's single payer advocates press ahead. SocialistWorker.org, March 16, 2010.

19. Merrick, A. States sink in benefits hole. *Wall Street Journal*, February 18, 2010: A4.
20. Denning L. Slump in tax revenue creates state of siege. *Wall Street Journal*, February 19, 2010: C10.
21. Sack, K, Pear, R. States consider Medicaid cuts as use grows. *New York Times*, February 19, 2010: A1.
22. Hennessy-Fiske, M, Gong Lin, R. L.A. County slashes doctors' reimbursement rate. *Los Angeles Times*, February 17, 2010.
23. Newton, C. Governor signs Ariz. budget-balancing bills. *The Arizona Republic*, March 18, 2010.
24. Sack, K. Medicaid payments shrink, more patients are abandoned. *New York Times*, March 16, 2010: A1.
25. Office of the Actuary, Centers for Medicare and Medicaid Services. Health spending projections through 2019. *Health Affairs*, February 4, 2010.
26. Woolhandler, S, Himmelstein, DU. Paying for national health insurance—and not getting it. *Health Affairs* 21 (4): 88-98, 2002.
27. Foster, RS. Estimated financial effects of the "Patient Protection and Affordable Care Act", as amended. Office of the Actuary of CMS. April 22, 2010.
28. Sirota, D. Progressive, liberal, what's the difference? *The Progressive Populist* 16 (8): 7, May 1, 2010.
29. Anderson, GF, Reinhardt, UW, Hussey, PI, Petrosyan, V. It's the prices, stupid:Why the United States is so different from other countries. *Health Affairs* 22 (3): 89-105, 2003.
30. Carroll, AE, Ackermann, RT. Support for national health insurance among U.S. physicians: Five years later. *Ann Intern Med* 1481: 566-7, 2008.
31. McCanne, D. Commenting on Op-Ed by William Pewen in *New York Times*, reference #6; (quote-of-the-day@mccanne.org), March 17, 2010.
32. Kaiser Family Foundation. Kaiser Health Tracking Poll. Publication $ 8067-C, April 22, 2010.
33. Hellander, I. International health systems for single payer advocates. The National Health Program Reader. Leadership Training Institute. Chicago, IL. Physicians for a National Health Program, October 24, 2008, pp 46-7.
34. Phillips, M. GOP candidates court seniors. *Wall Street Journal*, April 22, 2010: A5.
35. Hacker, JS. *The Divided Welfare State: The Battle Over Public and Private Social Benefits in the United States*. Cambridge, MA: Cambridge University Press. 2002, p 329.
36. Mullins, B. Senators seek cash as they mull rules. *Wall Street Journal*, April 21, 2010: A4.
37. Zinn, H. *A Power Governments Cannot Suppress*. San Francisco. City Lights Books. 2007, p 33.
38. Burns, JF. Conservatives in Britain retake political power. *New York Times*, May 12, 2010: A1.

39. Armstrong, P. Socialized healthcare: The 'untouchable' of UK politics. CNN, May 5, 2010.

40. Emerson, RW. As cited in Atkinson, B. (Ed) *The Essential Writings of Ralph Waldo Emerson.* New York. The Modern Library. Random House, 2000: xvi-xvii.

41. Himmelfarb, R. *Catastrophic Politics: The Rise and Fall of the Medicare Coverage Act of 1988.* University Park. Pennsylvania State University Press, 1995, p. 80.

42. de Tocqueville, A. As cited in Christakis, NA, Fowler, JH. *Connected: The Surprising Power of Our Social Networks and How They Shape Our Lives.* New York. Little, Brown and Company. 2009, p 293.

43. Giroux, HA. Reclaiming public values in the age of casino capitalism. *Truthout*, December 23, 2009.

44. Perkins, J. *Hoodwinked: An Economic Hit Man Reveals Why the World Financial Markets Imploded—and What We Need to Do to Remake Them.* New York. Broadway Books, 2009, pp 202-3.

45. Hedges, C. Ralph Nader was right about Barack Obama. *Truthdig*, March 1, 2010.

46. Adams, S. As cited in Hightower, J. *Swim Against the Current: Even a Dead Fish Can Go with the Flow.* Hoboken, NJ. John Wiley & Sons, Inc, 2008, p 193.

47. Christakis, NA, Fowler, JH. *Connected: The Surprising Power of Our Social Networks and How They Shape Our Lives.* New York. Little, Brown and Company. 2009, pp 28-31.

48. Nichols, J. MVPs of 2009. Most Valuable Think Tank. *The Nation* 290:2, January 11/18, 2010, p. 19.

49. Personal communication, Dr. Robert Stone, March 14, 2010.

50. Zinn, H. as cited in Rothschild, M. Thank you, Howard. *The Progressive* 74 (3): 4-5, 2010.

Index

About the Author

John Geyman, M.D. is Professor Emeritus of Family Medicine at the University of Washington School of Medicine in Seattle, where he served as Chairman of the Department of Family Medicine from 1976 to 1990. As a family physician with over 25 years in academic medicine, he has also practiced in rural communities for 13 years. He was the founding editor of *The Journal of Family Practice* (1973 to 1990) and the editor of *The Journal of the American Board of Family Practice* (1990 to 2003). His most recent books are *Health Care in America: Can Our Ailing System Be Healed?* (Butterworth-Heinemann, 2002), *The Corporate Transformation of Health Care: Can the Public Interest Still Be Served?* (Springer Publishing Company, 2004), *Falling Through the Safety Net: Americans Without Health Insurance* (Common Courage Press, 2005), *Shredding the Social Contract: The Privatization of Medicare* (Common Courage Press, 2006), *The Corrosion of Medicine: Can the Profession Reclaim its Moral Legacy?* (Common Courage Press, 2007), *Do Not Resuscitate: Why the Insurance Industry is Dying, and How We Must Replace It* (Common Courage Press, 2008), and *The Cancer Generation: Baby Boomers Facing a Perfect Storm* (Common Courage Press, 2009). Dr. Geyman served as President of Physicians for a National Health Program from 2005 to 2007 and is a member of the Institute of Medicine.

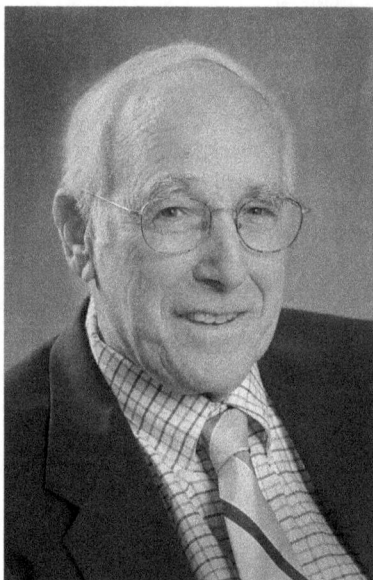

www.ingramcontent.com/pod-product-compliance
Lightning Source LLC
Chambersburg PA
CBHW031919190326
41519CB00007B/352